THE IVF JOURNAL

THE IVF
JOURNAL

The Solution for Managing Practitioners, Tests,
Medications, Appointments, Procedures, Finances,
and the Emotional Aspects of Your Journey

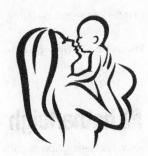

STEPHANIE FRY

Hatherleigh Press is committed to preserving and protecting the natural resources of the earth. Environmentally responsible and sustainable practices are embraced within the company's mission statement.

Visit us at www.hatherleighpress.com and register online for free offers, discounts, special events, and more.

The IVF Journal

Library of Congress Cataloging-in-Publication Data is available.
ISBN: 978-1-57826-492-6

DISCLAIMER
This book does not give legal or medical advice. Always consult your doctor, lawyer, and other professionals. The ideas and suggestions contained in this book are not intended as a substitute for consulting with a physician. All matters regarding your health require medical supervision.

Cover and Interior Design by Carolyn Kasper

Printed in the United States

10 9 8 7 6 5 4 3 2 1

hatherleigh
www.hatherleighpress.com

For Millie

CONTENTS

SECTION II:
CLINIC AND MEDICAL PROVIDERS

Chapter 4: YOUR MEDICAL TEAM:
A NEW KIND OF VILLAGE

SECTION III:
FINANCES

Chapter 5: FINANCES AND IVF:
LAYING THE GROUNDWORK

SECTION V:
WAIT AND RESULTS

SECTION VI:
SUPPORT FOR MIND AND BODY

SECTION VII:
MULTIPLE CYCLES

CLOSING

A NOTE FROM THE AUTHOR

Dear Readers,

In-vitro fertilization (IVF) is an incredibly personal experience that will require you to take in a great deal of new, constantly changing information. As such, no two individuals will experience IVF quite the same way. Each one of us will have different feelings and experiences throughout the process; therefore, I am not going to presume to tell you how the medical and emotional aspects of IVF will affect you personally. What I *can* and *will* do is offer information, advice, and guidance to help you along the way. I created *The IVF Journal* for a number of reasons. First and foremost, I wanted to keep my head above water during my own IVF experience. For years I existed within the constant storm of information and emotions that makes up the world of infertility and IVF. Eventually, one thing became clear: in order to survive the situation, I would need to take hold of the things that I *could* control, such as knowledge about my specific situation, my body, my cycles, and my feelings. The original IVF Journal began as a notebook, with a few simple lists and charts, and evolved slowly over many cycles into an organizational system that not only helped me to survive, but allowed me to thrive in the oftentimes challenging and overwhelming situations I found myself in.

    The IVF Journal has been invaluable as a means to reduce stress during my cycles. It has helped me to focus on my treatment, as well as to view the experience objectively, in a positive, productive manner, and has therefore helped me to better understand myself and the entire process. Tracking, documenting, and organizing the vast amount of information involved in the IVF process has saved me countless hours, headaches, as well as money. Having a tangible companion to turn to every time I head out to an appointment, have a question, or receive new information has been a great comfort.

The IVF Journal allowed me to have an open and educated dialogue with my medical providers, my husband, my family, and perhaps most importantly, myself. It has given me a greater understanding of the connections between physical and emotional responses, and has provided an outlet for my fears and frustrations. Understand that you cannot control what is going to happen in a cycle; but you *can* better understand what might happen, what *has* happened, and what your options are for moving forward.

My hope is that *The IVF Journal* becomes a positive part of your IVF experience; one that helps to reduce stress and allows you to better understand your specific situation. I hope it will help you to ask informed questions, make informed decisions and become a more confident participant in your medical care. I hope it will provide you with a personalized way to organize, store, and evaluate the information that is important and relevant to you.

As it has for me, I hope using *The IVF Journal* makes your journey clearer and less difficult. I hope it provides you with a sense of calm, clarity, and control by providing you with the opportunity and the tools to fully participate in a process that can often feel very chaotic and beyond your control. I hope it provides a productive way to pass the time while you wait for a cycle to start, or as you pass the hours in waiting room after waiting room. I hope it becomes something positive to focus on as you wait for the next instruction call, administer the next shot, get through the retrieval, wait for the fertilization report, go through the transfer and, of course, as you wait and wait for the results.

The IVF Journal is *your* book; not mine, and not your doctors'. Nor is it the latest and greatest in advice on how to get and stay pregnant. This book is meant to serve as your guide, one that will allow you to write your own story, on your own terms, in your own words.

Throughout this journey, remember: just attempting a cycle—whether canceled or completed, negative or positive—is a feat that takes strength, courage and an amazing amount of discipline and time. All that you endure, and the massive personal and family effort that goes into an IVF cycle, is always something to take great pride in.

With hope,

Stephanie Fry

Chapter 1

HOW TO USE THE IVF JOURNAL

FOR MOST WOMEN undergoing IVF, the process is an all-encompassing and life-altering experience. It involves multiple practitioners and contacts, a significant financial investment, and a seemingly endless stream of medications, tests, appointments, and procedures. It is the subject of thousands of books, articles, blogs, and websites. Stress, long waits, questions, excitement, hopes, uncertainties, and worries are just part of the territory.

The IVF Journal will help you to better manage the entire process by providing a place for you to organize contacts, information, and resources. It will help you to prepare emotionally, financially, and logistically; it provides systems for tracking and recording treatments, results, responses, and progress. It allows you to explore, define and manage your personal IVF journey (both emotionally and physically) in your own words and in your own way.

Using this journal can ease your stress and help you make the most of your treatment allowing you to have a more positive IVF experience, no matter what the outcome.

It is okay to admit that going through IVF is a big deal! It is exciting, complicated, challenging, expensive, and important. And just like any other major life event, this time of your life deserves to be—and will be—well served by a little extra attention, organization, and preparation.

YOUR BOOK, YOUR RULES

The IVF Journal is *your* book and *you* decide how to use it. This is not a "my way or the highway" situation; rather, it is more like a big suggestion box has just landed in your lap and you can take from it what you need. If something doesn't work for you, change it. If you don't need, want, or like a certain page or section, skip it. Wouldn't it be great if this tactic could be applied in everyday life when dealing with infertility? Unfortunately you can't easily rework the pages of life, but you can certainly decide how you use this book.

For instance: if you are not covered by insurance, then by all means skip those worksheets. If you want nothing to do with complementary therapies, you can ignore that content without a trace of guilt. Chart your follicle growth but not your hormone levels, use the Tax Planner or don't; log your two-week wait symptoms and your emotions and skip the journaling, or vice versa. It's up to you.

Not only that, but you also decide how often to use *The IVF Journal*. When you are in a cycle, there may be days when you just don't feel like making entries. Just toss your results and instructions in the book, maybe jot down a few notes, and wait until you're in the mood. Use the book all day long, or make your entries once a day, once a week, when you have an appointment, or whenever feels right for you. Infertility can come with a lot of guilt; using *The IVF Journal* should not add to that burden.

USING THE IVF JOURNAL FOR THIRD-PARTY REPRODUCTION CYCLES

For patients who are using third-party reproduction, please understand that, while *The IVF Journal* is written from the perspective of a two-partner cycle, it can be easily adapted for use in third-party reproduction. If you are doing IVF using donor eggs, donor sperm, donor embryos, or a gestational carrier, you can still use the charts effectively; just make notes and adjustments as needed.

A FEW THINGS TO KEEP IN MIND

Throughout your treatment and as you use *The IVF Journal*, consider the following:

DON'T PLAN, PREPARE. Because there are so many variables in IVF, you simply will not be able to plan the exact timing, outcome, or experience of an IVF cycle—but you should always be prepared for one.

The old adage of "hope for the best, plan for the worst, and expect the unexpected" will come in handy here. Your journey will be easier if you get comfortable with the fact that you can't control what is going to happen *during* the cycle, as it is impossible to have everything figured out ahead of time. What you can control is how you prepare for a cycle. Arming yourself with facts, information, systems, options, and ideas before you get started allows you to better cope with any and all eventualities.

DON'T COMPARE—ONE SIZE DOES <u>NOT</u> FIT ALL. Do not worry about comparing your cycle to anyone else's or to what is considered "normal." In the land of IVF there *is* no "normal." Clinics and physicians cycle and test differently, and use different systems and milestones for each patient based on their specific diagnoses. If you want to gauge your levels, ask your reproductive endocrinologist (RE) what they are looking for in your specific case.

Don't worry, or assume something is wrong if there are things mentioned in this book that your doctor or nurses have not addressed, or if you are being tested for something that is not listed here. *The IVF Journal* is designed to cover many different types of IVF cycles, so it is highly unlikely that each situation will apply to every person. For instance: in the Clinic and Medical Providers section (see page 31), smaller clinics may have only one or two points of contact whereas larger ones will have dedicated contact information for multiple individuals. Similarly, some patients require only one or two types of medication, while others require more. Just make adjustments as needed and ask your RE if you have any questions about the tests you are (or are not) receiving.

GO TO THE SOURCE. If you have any medical questions or concerns (and you will hear me repeat this often) talk to your RE or their staff. They are your absolute best source of information. And remember that use of the Internet and/or books about IVF (including this one) are *not* intended to replace medical treatment or to help you self-diagnose. The Web has hundreds (if not thousands) of blogs, chat rooms, message boards, and websites dedicated to infertility and IVF. If you are so inclined, these sites can be wonderful resources, but always be mindful of the source and use your common sense. Never let information from an unverified, un-moderated, insensitive, or biased source upset you or trump your doctor's advice.

DO WHAT FEELS RIGHT. As you go through IVF treatment you are likely to come across loads of different types of tips, advice, and complementary therapy options. As you encounter and consider these things, always remember that while there are plenty of experts out there, there is only one expert on *you*. Make sure you listen to your heart and your body throughout the entire process. Whether it is a new diet, a new mind-body technique, advice on how much you should exercise, or what vitamins to take, if something you are doing doesn't feel right, honor that feeling. Know that while it may have worked great for someone else, that doesn't mean it is right for you.

KNOW WHEN TO SAY WHEN. Make sure that you consider how much information is enough for you. For some people, too many details about their cycles can feel overwhelming. Make sure you are comfortable with the level of information you are receiving from your providers. If you do not want specifics on your cycle, such as follicle growth details or regular hormone level updates, let your providers know. Similarly, tell them if you want all the information available, and know that you can change your mind at any time.

MAKE TIME TO LEARN THE BASICS. *The IVF Journal* assumes that you have been (or are in the process of being) diagnosed and that you are under the care of a physician who has helped you determine that IVF is the best course of treatment for you. It also assumes that you have a basic understanding of an IVF cycle, as well as the second language that is ART, IVF, and the like. The IVF Basics section (see page 9) and the Glossary (see page 163) will get you started, but because there are so many possible infertility diagnoses, causes, and treatment plans, you should make sure you have a good understanding of your specific situation. For most patients IVF is uncharted territory, and having a deeper understanding of all aspects of the process will help you to cycle with confidence and surety. The Diagnoses Worksheet and Treatment Worksheet in Chapter 3 can provide space to explore this (with your doctor's help).

KNOW THAT IVF TREATMENT IS ALWAYS EVOLVING. New tests, medical devices, procedures, and medications are being put into to use every day. This constant innovation provides advances in infertility treatment and can mean more successful IVF cycles. It also means that you can expect to have more choice (and more information to process) when it comes to your treatment. In the coming months and years patients can expect a growing "menu" of ancillary treatments, procedures, and medical devices which will include everything from genetic testing options to new technologies for viewing embryos in the lab to new medications and more.

All of this innovation may affect how many and what providers you interact with, your financials, and your treatment plan so as often as possible *The IVF Journal* has included space for "other" options and notes pages so you will have space to document any new innovations not currently listed.

SECTION OVERVIEW

The IVF Journal consists of seven sections, most with multiple chapters. Each chapter includes instructions on how to use the calendars, charts, logs, and worksheets contained in that chapter. Because the physical, emotional, and financial aspects of an IVF cycle are inevitably intertwined, I recommend you review all the sections applicable to your situation *before* you begin; but, if you want to jump right into a certain section, go right ahead; I certainly can't ask a woman in an IVF cycle to wait for anything else, so have at it! Just know that you can always reference this quick guide as you go.

SECTION I: IVF BASICS

This introductory section covers basic information about IVF treatment and how best to prepare for it. It includes the medical phases of a cycle and possible risks (including cycle cancelation and outcomes) as well as a basic overview of some of the general causes of infertility.

SECTION II: CLINICS AND MEDICAL PROVIDERS

This section covers IVF clinics, physicians, pharmacies, and other medical providers. It will be your go-to resource for names, phone numbers, emails, addresses, and provider policies.

SECTION III: FINANCES

This section covers every financial aspect of your cycle—cycle pricing, payment, and financing options, as well as expense tracking, insurance, and taxes.

SECTION IV: IVF CYCLE

This section covers the actual IVF cycle process, including schedules and timing, medications, egg retrieval, embryo growth, and transfer.

SECTION V: WAIT AND RESULTS

This section helps you to plan for—and survive—the end of the long road that is IVF: the two-week wait and the results.

SECTION VI: SUPPORT FOR MIND AND BODY

This section will help you support yourself emotionally and physically during your IVF treatment by creating your own personal support network. It also helps you navigate complementary therapies and manage your emotions by practicing self-awareness.

SECTION VII: MULTIPLE CYCLES

The IVF Journal is designed to cover one cycle; but, because many patients cycle more than once, this section is dedicated to multiple cycles, offering strategies and advice for longer term treatment and allowing for comparison of up to four IVF cycles, side by side. It also covers frozen embryo transfers (FETs).

SECTION I
IVF BASICS

Chapter 2

UNDERSTANDING IVF: A CYCLE IN FIVE PHASES

BEFORE YOU BEGIN preparing for IVF it is crucial that you have a basic understanding of the process. By definition, in-vitro fertilization (IVF) is the joining of a woman's egg and a man's sperm in a laboratory dish to create a viable embryo. During the process, eggs are retrieved from your ovaries and fertilized by sperm in a lab. The fertilized egg becomes an embryo, which is placed in your uterus where it will hopefully implant. That is IVF in a nutshell; and while all cycles are different, they do follow a basic system. To really be prepared for your specific situation, you will need to dig a little deeper and understand the way a cycle actually works. In order to do this, it can be helpful to break down your cycle into its five phases:

1. Pre-Cycle

2. Stimulation

3. Egg Retrieval and Semen Collection

4. Fertilization and Embryo Growth

5. Embryo Transfer and Results

What follows is a basic description of those phases. If you are interested in more detailed medical and scientific information, you can ask your team at the clinic for medical reference books or refer to the Organizations listed on pages 159–161. You can also refer to the Glossary on page 163 for more detailed definitions of tests, procedures, and medications.

PHASE ONE: PRE-CYCLE

Your pre-cycle phase marks the start of your treatment and usually lasts a few weeks. In this phase, your body is being prepared for treatment, and you will likely have multiple appointments and tests. If you haven't already, you will soon receive schedules, instructions, medications, and paperwork from your clinic and other providers. Most patients will also begin taking some medications during this phase as well.

The pre-cycle phase usually includes some, if not all, of the following tests and medications:

- A sonohysterography and/or a hysteroscopy test may be used to view your uterine cavity and determine if there are any issues that may interfere with treatment. For similar reasons, and to determine the shape and depth of your uterine cavity, your treatment plan may also include a mock-transfer, a sort of "practice round," to help ensure a smoother embryo transfer.

- A semen analysis is sometimes done shortly before the start of a treatment cycle (even if earlier tests showed no problems) to ensure that sperm quality and counts have not changed.

- In most, if not all cases, you and your partner will both receive infectious disease screening including tests for HIV, hepatitis B, hepatitis C and, in some cases, chlamydia. You will likely also need to provide an up-to-date physical from your primary care physician.

- Many patients take oral contraceptives or birth control pills during this phase. This is to make sure things will start at the proper time and can help to regulate irregular cycles; this can also help prevent ovarian cysts, which can disrupt or delay a cycle. Some patients, particularly those with ovulation issues, may begin taking progesterone or other hormones at this time as well.

- Suppression medications are often given during this phase to ensure that you do not ovulate too early. There are multiple types and lengths of suppression medications, the two most common being a GnRH agonist (which is usually started during the pre-cycle phase) and a GnRH antagonist (which is given in phase two, after stimulation has started).

- Ovarian reserve testing may be performed to evaluate your remaining egg supply. There are numerous ovarian reserve tests available and since none of the tests are perfect, your RE may use a combination of tests to gain a better understanding of your remaining egg supply which can help predict how your ovaries will respond to fertility medication. Many clinics use what is commonly referred to as FSH or Day 3 testing to measure the follicle-stimulating hormone level (FSH) in your blood on day three of your menstrual cycle. Others use an AMH Fertility Test which can be done on any day of your cycle by measuring Anti Mullerian Hormones. Still others use a vaginal ultrasound to perform an antral follicle count. On day three of your cycle you may also receive a baseline pelvic ultrasound, which examines your ovaries to make sure there are no cysts or other issues that may interfere with your cycle. These tests, if employed, will usually mark the close of your pre-cycle phase and the beginning of phase two of your cycle: stimulation.

PHASE TWO: STIMULATION

Stimulation is all about egg production. During stimulation you may end up taking any number of medications based on your needs, but the basic purpose is to "stimulate" the ovaries to produce multiple follicles or eggs, instead of the single egg that is normally produced each month. Multiple eggs are needed because not all eggs fertilize, and of those that do, not all embryos will develop normally after fertilization. To stimulate egg production, you will take a series of injections of FSH, or follicle-stimulating hormone. It is also possible that during stimulation you will still be taking some suppression medications, as well as several other medicines that you started during your pre-cycle phase.

During stimulation, you will have regular trans-vaginal ultrasounds and blood work done to check your ovaries and hormone levels. This is also referred to as "monitoring." Monitoring is frequent, usually every other day. Based on the results of your monitoring tests you will receive instructions to either adjust your medications or keep the levels the same. You will also receive information on how many follicles are developing on each ovary. Keep in mind that ultrasounds are not always exactly accurate, and there is not always a mature egg in every follicle. Information about the exact number of eggs will not be verified until after your egg retrieval.

Stimulation can last anywhere from a few days to two weeks, and ends with what is commonly called a "trigger shot." The trigger shot is a dose of medication (given by injection) that induces ovulation and helps your eggs mature, so that they can be ready for fertilization. Another term you might hear for this shot is a HCG or human chorionic gonadotropin shot. Your reproductive endocrinologist (RE) will use the information available from your blood work and ultrasound monitoring to determine the exact day and time for you to take the trigger shot.

Your trigger shot signifies the end of phase two, and your eggs will usually be retrieved 34 to 36 hours after the trigger shot.

PHASE THREE: EGG RETRIEVAL AND SEMEN COLLECTION

The third phase starts the procedural phase of your cycle. You will be asked to arrive at your clinic at a specified time on the day of your egg retrieval. Most patients will be instructed not to eat or drink anything that morning, and there may be other restrictions, such as not wearing perfumes or scented lotions, which can interfere with laboratory environments. Some larger clinics have a hospital-type setting, where you and your partner will don scrubs and hairnets for the egg retrieval procedure; others will have a less clinical atmosphere. Some patients are surprised to learn that their RE does not actually perform their egg retrieval and/or transfer procedure. This is because many clinics use a system where members of the practice work on rotation. If that is how your clinic operates, the RE who performs your retrieval will be determined by that rotation. Barring any last minute changes you can ask your nurse or patient coordinator who will be performing your retrieval (and transfer) ahead of time.

Semen is either collected at home (if your home is not too far away) and brought to the clinic at the time of retrieval; or it will be collected on-site right before the egg retrieval procedure. It will then be prepared for fertilization by being "washed" (meaning the sperm is separated from the seminal fluid) and prepared for fertilization.

Egg retrieval, medically known as follicular aspiration, is a minor surgery that removes the eggs from your body. It is an outpatient procedure that uses ultrasound images to help your RE insert a thin needle through your vagina and then into the ovary and follicles containing the eggs. The needle is connected to a suction device, which pulls the eggs out of each follicle, one at a time.

In most cases an anesthesiologist administers intravenous medications (sedatives and pain relievers), so patients sleep through the procedure and feel nothing. Some patients may experience cramping and discomfort after the surgery, but this usually goes away within a day or two.

The procedure is repeated on each ovary and only takes about 30 minutes. When you wake up, you will be told how many eggs were retrieved. After your eggs are retrieved, they are transferred to a lab where they are kept under special conditions.

On the day of egg retrieval, most patients begin taking progesterone in the form of oral tablets, injections, or vaginal suppositories. Progesterone helps prepare your body for a pregnancy and, among other things, helps the lining of your uterus get ready to receive embryos, which happens in the next phase: fertilization and embryo growth.

PHASE FOUR: FERTILIZATION AND EMBRYO GROWTH

After your retrieval, your partner's semen is placed in a culture medium along with your eggs, in the hopes that a sperm will enter, or fertilize, your egg. A culture medium is a nutrient substance that is used to cultivate microorganisms. It provides ideal, specialized conditions for the egg and sperm and later the resulting embryo.

If your RE thinks the chances of fertilization are low, or if you have sperm quality or quantity issues, a technique called ICSI (intracytoplasmic sperm injection) may be used to fertilize your eggs. During ICSI, a single healthy sperm is injected directly into each mature egg. ICSI is also often used if fertilization attempts during prior IVF cycles have failed.

After fertilization, the resulting embryos are placed in small dishes or tubes containing another culture medium which resembles the fluid found in your fallopian tubes and uterus and is designed to help the embryos develop. Once embryos begin to develop, they are placed into incubators, which provide controlled lighting, temperature, and humidity.

In most cases you will receive a call the day after your retrieval to let you know how many eggs were successfully fertilized, and how many then divided to become embryos. Over the next few days, the embryos are viewed regularly to make sure they are growing properly.

Before transfer, some patients may have genetic testing or screening performed on their embryos. Currently the two most commonly used tests are pre-implantation genetic diagnosis (PGD) or comparative genomic hybridization (CGH) testing.

PGD, which is usually performed on day 3 or 5 before transfer, is a specialized genetic test used to evaluate one cell, or cells, from an embryo for chromosome abnormalities and/or diseases due to a single gene mutation. Similarly, CGH testing is also performed on embryos before transfer, but this procedure tests for a broader range of chromosomal abnormalities, so that the embryos with the most normal chromosomal profile can be selected for transfer. These tests are not offered at all clinics and may be expensive, but can be helpful in diagnosing the cause of failed IVF cycles, repeated miscarriages, and unexplained infertility. Genetic testing including Carrier Screening, which tests parents for genetic disorders before starting IVF, is also helpful for high risk patients who run the risk of passing on genetic disorders such as sickle cell anemia or cystic fibrosis.

If you have specific factors, such as advanced maternal age, previous failed IVF attempts, or other embryo and implantation issues, your RE might recommend assisted hatching. This is a technique where a hole is made in the membrane of the embryo to help it "hatch" out of its outer shell and implant in the lining of your uterus. If employed, assisted hatching is done just before embryo transfer.

Whether or not you are using ICSI, genetic testing, or assisted hatching, the final phase of your cycle, the transfer and results phase, will come directly after fertilization and embryo growth, about three to five days after your egg retrieval.

PHASE FIVE: EMBRYO TRANSFER AND RESULTS

Your treatment plan will likely specify ahead of time if you are to have a three-day or a five-day transfer. A three-day transfer simply means your embryos will be placed in your uterus after three days of lab growth, while a five-day transfer means they will be allowed to grow in the lab setting for two more days, making a total of five days. It is not unusual to hear of a four-day transfer but three or five days remains the norm.

Keep in mind that scheduled transfer days can and often do change. For instance, if your treatment plan specifies a five-day transfer, but on day two the clinic's embryologist makes a determination that a three-day transfer is preferable, they will change your transfer to a three-day. This can happen in the other direction as well; many patients scheduled for a three-day transfer will end up having a five-day transfer instead. The decision on which day to transfer hinges on multiple factors and contrary to what many patients think there is no proof that either system (day 3 or 5) is preferable or has statistically better results. If you have questions about what is preferable speak with your RE about your specific case and treatment plan.

On the day of your transfer, the embryos that look "the best" are selected for transfer. Determining which embryos are best is a process often referred to as embryo grading. Embryo grades are usually based on the number of cells an embryo has on a certain day and how fragmented (or broken up) they are. Embryo grading varies widely from clinic to clinic (some use letter grades and others numbers) and is very subjective, so much so that embryologists often must make educated guesses based on their past experience. Due to its subjectivity and the fact that there is no set standard for grading embryos, it is highly recommended that you understand and document how your specific clinic grades and selects embryos. There is space on page 39 for you to do so.

When you arrive for your transfer, you will likely have a conversation with your RE (or the one on duty that day) or your clinics embryologist about the quality of your embryos and the amount (if not pre-determined) to transfer. In many clinics, you will be able to see your embryos on a big screen and may even get a picture of them to take home.

Right before your transfer you might be given a mild sedative to help you relax, and you may be asked to drink water so your bladder will be full during transfer. Having a full bladder can be uncomfortable, but not painful, and allows your RE the best access to your uterus.

Your RE (or a nurse) will insert a catheter into your vagina, through your cervix and into your uterus. For those who have had them, this is similar to an intrauterine insemination. Next, a syringe containing your embryo(s) is attached to the end of the catheter, and the fluid, along with the embryos, is pushed into your uterus.

At this point you are almost finished. The waiting period after transfer varies, and some clinics require bed rest, but many do not, and after as little as a 15-minute rest you will be on your way. If you have extra embryos that meet your clinic's qualifications, they will be frozen to be transferred at a later date, if necessary. You can ask about this process or wait to be notified by your clinic about how many embryos "made it to freeze."

You will continue taking the progesterone support you started after egg retrieval until your pregnancy test, which measures the level of HCG in your blood and will be done 10–14 days after your embryo transfer. If positive, the test is usually repeated a few days later to make sure your levels are rising adequately, and you will likely be required to continue progesterone and any other support medications you are taking for several weeks or longer. If the test is negative you will be told to stop taking progesterone and your cycle will be complete.

RISKS, CANCELATIONS, AND OUTCOMES

Like all medical procedures, there are some risks associated with IVF treatment. You may also be surprised to learn that an IVF cycle, once underway, can be canceled. And, as many people are also surprised to learn, your results are not always negative or positive: there *are* gray areas, and positive cycles do not always equal a full-term pregnancy. These risks, while not the norm, are worth reviewing so you will not be blindsided should one of them occur.

RISKS

The risks below (and others associated with IVF) have undoubtedly been discussed with you in more detail by your medical providers, but it is worthwhile to review the more common risks of IVF.

- Fertility drugs can cause ovarian hyperstimulation syndrome (OHSS). If you develop OHSS, your ovaries may become swollen and painful, and you may experience abdominal pain, bloating, nausea, vomiting, and diarrhea. These symptoms can last a few days or up to a week and be the cause of cycle cancelation.

- IVF increases the risk of multiple pregnancies, especially if more than one embryo is transferred to your uterus.

- Rarely, there can be egg retrieval procedure complications, and of course there are risks associated with general anesthesia and other sedative medications.

CANCELATIONS

There are quite a few things that can disrupt or drastically change the course of an IVF cycle. A canceled cycle, understandably, can be shocking and difficult for patients who have cause to experience one. The Clinic Operations Worksheets in Chapter 4 will guide you through figuring out your clinic's specific criteria, but some common causes of a cycle being canceled are:

- Ovarian cysts detected before or during stimulation

- Inadequate number of follicles developing

- Pre-mature ovulation

- Too many follicles developing/OHSS (ovarian hyperstimulation syndrome)

And even after retrieval, other things can happen during the fertilization process that may cause cycle cancellation:

- Follicles do not contain mature eggs

- Fertilization of the eggs may fail to happen

- Eggs (some or all) may fertilize abnormally, resulting in abnormal embryos

- Embryos may fail to develop (or divide) or arrest (stop developing)

OUTCOMES

A positive IVF cycle does not always equal a full-term pregnancy, and while positive results that come with little hope for a live birth are not the norm, it is good sense to be aware of all potential outcomes so that there will be no surprises. If you find yourself in one of these situations you may be faced with more waiting, testing, and some tough decisions. Make sure you ask your providers for information and resources, so you can understand what is happening. The best method for finding ways to cope and figure out your options for moving forward is to be educated.

ECTOPIC PREGNANCY. About 2 percent of women who use in-vitro fertilization will have an ectopic pregnancy. An ectopic pregnancy occurs when a fertilized egg implants in the wrong place. It can be outside of the uterus or in a fallopian tube.

BLIGHTED OVUM. A blighted ovum, also known as an anembryonic pregnancy, happens when a fertilized egg attaches itself to the uterine wall and forms a pregnancy sac but the embryo does not develop.

CHEMICAL PREGNANCY. In chemical pregnancies, which are common in natural conception as well as with IVF treatment, a miscarriage happened very early in the pregnancy—oftentimes before the five-week mark, or even as early as within a week after your transfer.

MISCARRIAGE. When the pregnancy develops further, to the point that ultrasound can confirm the existence of the pregnancy, a miscarriage can still occur. The rate of miscarriage for women who get pregnant through IVF is about 15 to 20 percent, about the same as women who conceive naturally.

INFERTILITY CAUSES: A BASIC OVERVIEW

Infertility and the resulting need for IVF can be caused by many factors, and every patient is different. A few potential causes of infertility are listed below. For more information on these or anything else you may be being treated for, you can talk to your providers or turn to one of the organizations listed on pages 159–161 for more information.

- Fallopian tube damage or blockage makes it difficult or impossible for an egg to be fertilized, or for an embryo to reach the uterus.

- Ovulation disorders, such as absent, infrequent, or irregular ovulation, means that no eggs are available for fertilization.

- Premature ovarian failure occurs when a women loses normal ovarian function before age 40, usually because the ovaries don't produce normal amounts of estrogen or release eggs regularly.

- Endometriosis is a condition that occurs when uterine tissue grows outside of the uterus and impairs the function of the ovaries, uterus, and fallopian tubes.

- PCOS, or polycystic ovary syndrome, is a common endocrine (or hormonal) disorder that impairs fertility among women of reproductive age.

- Uterine fibroids are benign tumors in the wall of the uterus that can interfere with implantation of the fertilized egg.

- Below-average sperm concentration, weak movement of sperm, or abnormalities in sperm size and shape can make it difficult or impossible for sperm to fertilize an egg.

- Unexplained infertility, which occurs in about 10–20 percent of patients, means no cause of infertility has been found.

- Other health conditions, such as celiac disease, thyroid disease (or disorder), cancer, and resulting treatments can cause infertility.

Again, this is just the tip of the iceberg of infertility causes, any of which can lead to the need for IVF. The best thing you can do to help you better understand your treatment is to learn about the cause of your infertility diagnoses. Space to do so is provided in the Diagnosis Worksheet on page 28.

Chapter 3

PREPPING FOR IVF

PREP TIPS FOR A SMOOTH CYCLE

Infertility treatment can be a bumpy road, stressful and full of surprises. Even when things go perfectly, for most patients the process involves uncharted territory and deserves preparation. Here are a few ways you can prepare for IVF and pave the way for a smoother cycle.

UNDERSTAND YOUR TREATMENT. The unknown is scary. The feeling that you are in the dark about your treatment can add greatly to the stress of an IVF cycle. Instead of fixating on "what-ifs" and "maybes" in a worrisome, stressful way, you can choose to focus on your cycle in a positive, productive manner, by making an effort to understand your diagnosis, treatment, and all possible outcomes *before* you begin your cycle. Understanding the phases of your treatment demystifies the cycle process and boosts your confidence as you move through your cycle. Being prepared for all possible outcomes means that you will be ready to handle anything that comes your way—good or bad.

SCHEDULE TIME FOR CHANGE AND BE READY TO WAIT. IVF cycles tend to follow a basic timeline, but even these steps are unpredictable by nature—each step of the cycle hinges on the next, so one change can have a ripple effect that plays havoc on your emotions *and* on your schedule. It helps to get into a flexible mindset before you begin. Have a few backup plans in place: If you think you will need short notice coverage at work or at home, have several options open to you, and be ready to alter your plans if need be. Never forget that IVF cycles involve lots of waiting! You'll wait for the cycle to start; you'll wait for appointments, instructions, test results, procedural results; and of course, you'll wait for the big news. In fact, you wait so much there is an entire chapter in this book dedicated to just that!

CONSIDER YOUR STRESS THRESHOLD. Whether it is a tough family situation, a difficult relationship or a big presentation at work, we all have certain situations that are more stressful than others. If possible, consider rescheduling any high stress events during your cycle. This is especially important during your first cycle as you can't be exactly sure how things will affect you. The benefits of staying calm and happy during a cycle may be enough to outweigh skipping a few events. You could also consider waiting a month for treatment if you have something big that cannot be moved.

ANTICIPATE TOUGH MOMENTS. Before you start your cycle, have a discussion with your doctor, partner, or other important people in your life about the possible reactions to the process, medications, procedures, and stress. Not everyone will be adversely affected by these things, but it never hurts to recognize and anticipate your physical and emotional responses. The fact is that you may be a little (or a lot) exhausted, short-tempered, cranky, or on edge. If you discuss this possibility, as well as potential causes and solutions beforehand, a tense moment can be more easily diffused with a gentle reminder that you knew tough moments might occur and are just a reaction to stress, medications, and exhaustion—or a combination of all three!

GET ORGANIZED. Create a cycle management center. It can be a shoebox, a drawer, a binder—any place where you can keep all your cycle information and documentation in one place. This way, when you have a question or want to find information quickly, you will know where to look. Begin by gathering everything you have pertaining to IVF and infertility. Include all of the information provided by your clinic, pharmacy, and other practitioners. Don't forget financial information and documentation, including any insurance policies, receipts, payment and fee schedules, and bills. Finally, add in any pamphlets, organization brochures, websites, and any other information you have on hand. Having a go-to spot is a lifesaver when you want (or need) to find something quickly.

THINK OF IVF AS A JOURNEY, NOT A DESTINATION. IVF treatment is not a fast process. The length of time from when you decide to cycle to the big results day can often take months, and in some cases extended treatment can last years. For many, IVF and infertility require endurance. I say this not to scare you but to prepare you, in case your journey turns out to take longer than expected. Think of it as a marathon, not a sprint; this way, you can better navigate the journey if you end up having a longer course. If you expect it to be brief, and your expectations are not met, coping and continuing with treatment can be very difficult.

CONSIDER YOUR PERSONAL NETWORK. If you have been trying to conceive for some time, it is likely that you are used to fielding questions about your reproductive status. However, during IVF you may find yourself in a new debate about how much to tell certain folks. Sharing the news that you are doing IVF can be cathartic and can be less stressful than keeping things a secret. Sharing means you also may find support in unexpected places and may gain more understanding from family, friends, bosses, and co-workers. But you should also consider that there may be some possible negative aspects to sharing as well. Sharing details can invite unwanted inquiries, advice, questions, and insensitive comments, and you may find yourself having to educate people about IVF when you don't want to. At the same time, you may learn things about people's religious and political views that you never wanted to know! Finally, perhaps the most difficult aspect of sharing IVF details is that you will also have to share the bad news if the results are negative. It can be much harder to explain a failed cycle than it is to explain that you are going through treatment. No matter what you decide, it is a good idea to keep the specific timing of your results to yourself; that way you can share the news, positive or negative, at your own pace.

HOW TO USE THIS CHAPTER

The first worksheets in this book cover your diagnosis and treatment plan. Completing these worksheets ahead of time will lay the foundation for a less stressful cycle by giving you a better understanding of the entire IVF cycle process as it relates to your specific situation.

Complete the Diagnosis Worksheet by having a conversation with your reproductive endocrinologist (RE). If you haven't already, ask for a detailed explanation of your diagnosis and its underlying cause. Keep in mind that about 15 to 20% of couples will have a diagnosis of "Unexplained Infertility." This means that the fertility tests are normal and that there is no easily identifiable cause. If this is the case you can ask if your recommended treatment plan might help shed light on the cause of your infertility, which is often the case.

You and your partner might have tried less invasive treatment options in the past, including fertility drugs and Intrauterine insemination (IUI). If so, make sure to discuss those treatments and their outcomes as well. Ask how the information gained from the past might help to explain your diagnosis and how it might affect current treatment recommendations.

Finally, ask your RE what treatment plan she or he recommends, based on your diagnoses. Make sure to ask if you will need any ancillary treatments, such as ICSI (intra-cytoplasmic sperm Injection) or assisted hatching (AH),, and why. It is also a good idea to discuss a long-term scenario. Specifically: If the recommended treatment doesn't work, what are your options?

Once you understand *why* you are having IVF, you can use the Treatment Worksheet to help you understand and document your actual treatment plan specifics. This worksheet is based on the five phases of an IVF cycle, which were outlined in Chapter 2. You should review and understand the phases before asking your doctor, nurse, or other clinic contacts to explain how each phase will work.

Begin at the top of the Treatment Worksheet by filling in the basics of your plan. Add the name of your protocol and check off what day transfer is planned for, along with any additional procedures or genetic or other testing that may be performed. Remember that treatment plans can change based on the results of each phase. If you do not start out needing additional treatments such as ICSI or AH, you can ask if there are any eventualities that may make them necessary. If you are undecided about ancillary treatments or tests, circle the question mark.

Below are a few questions you can ask about each cycle phase that, if answered ahead of time, can help you understand what is happening as you move through the cycle:

- What will happen in each phase of the cycle, and what types of medications will I take during each phase?

- What is the goal? Or, what are we hoping to achieve in each phase? What would be a good response? A poor one?

- If my response in any given phase is poor, how will my treatment plan be adjusted?

- What potential physical or emotional side effects might I have to the medications and procedures in each phase?

The Treatment Worksheet ends with a box dedicated to Embryo Transfer Information. The decision regarding how many embryos to transfer is highly personal and can be controversial, so it is a good idea to discuss how many embryos you plan to transfer ahead of time. This decision is usually based on multiple factors including diagnosis, prior treatment outcomes, number of available eggs and embryos, and maternal age. Most clinics follow specific guidelines relating to how many embryos can be transferred, and many recommend single embryo transfers. They do this because while transferring multiple embryos may raise your chances of success, it also raises your risk of multiple pregnancies and resulting complications.

Here are a few questions you can ask so that you will have time to process the information you may need to make decisions about embryo transfer later in your cycle:

- Based on my diagnosis and age, how many embryos do you recommend I transfer?

- How will the number of embryos transferred affect my chances for success?

- How will that same number affect my risk of multiple pregnancies?

Once you have completed these worksheets, you should have a good understanding of your diagnosis and treatment, which is the absolute best way to start a cycle.

Diagnosis Overview and Information:

_____

_____

_____

_____

_____

_____

_____

_____

Past Treatments and Outcomes:

_____

_____

_____

_____

_____

Recommended Treatment Based on Diagnosis

_____

_____

_____

_____

_____

TREATMENT WORKSHEET

Protocol: _____

Planned Transfer Day: 3: _____   5: _____   Other: _____

Planned Procedures and Testing: ICSI: Y / N / ?   AH: Y / N / ?   Other: _____

Genetic Testing: Y / N / ?   Type: _____

Phase 1: Pre-Cycle

Phase 2: Stimulation

Phase 3: Egg Retrieval and Semen Collection

Phase 4: Fertilization and Embryo Growth

Phase 5: Embryo Transfer and Results

Embryo Transfer Information

DIAGNOSIS AND TREATMENT NOTES

_____

_____

_____

_____

_____

_____

_____

_____

_____

_____

_____

_____

_____

_____

_____

_____

_____

_____

_____

_____

_____

_____

SECTION II
CLINIC AND MEDICAL PROVIDERS

Chapter 4

YOUR MEDICAL TEAM: A NEW KIND OF VILLAGE

I T IS OFTEN said it takes a village to raise a child. When you start to undergo IVF, you will soon learn it also takes a village to make one! Somewhere between the realization that you may not be able to become pregnant naturally and the start of your cycle, you will start to notice that you are on a first name basis not only with your reproductive endocrinologist (RE) but also with your Nurse Coordinator, multiple ultrasound techs, your mail-order pharmacist, and maybe even the barista who opens your local coffee shop each morning. This, my friend, is your baby-making village. My advice is to get to know them, and get to know them well. Figure out who does what, how they do it and how to contact them when the need arises.

Having basic information at your fingertips (hours of operation, phone numbers, locations, and directions) means you don't have to spend your precious mental energy searching for basics when you are in the middle of your cycle. It takes only a little bit of legwork to determine the closest, least expensive, least stressful options available to you, but this information is worth its weight in gold and can save you time, money, and headaches in the long run.

It is equally as important to understand provider policies and procedures. Understanding the way your clinic, pharmacy, and other providers operate, communicate, and interact can help to eliminate surprises and minimize stress. When questions arise, you will know where to look for the answers, and if you can't find them, you will know who to ask and how to reach them. Finally, asking simple questions about the way a clinic operates really helps you to understand your treatment and know what to expect during your cycle.

HOW TO USE THIS CHAPTER

The information you need to complete the worksheets in this chapter, while straight-forward and fairly easy to find, is also *extremely* important, as it will likely be referenced over and over again throughout your cycle. If collecting the information and asking questions feels overwhelming or uncomfortable, get your partner involved by putting them in charge of contacting and documenting your contacts and their information.

Start with your infertility clinic, as it will be the driving force behind your cycle. Know that your RE and their team do much more than just administer your cycle; they carefully plan, execute, and constantly update your medications, protocol, and sched-ule based on your specific diagnosis and current testing. They are also the all-import-ant messengers during the process. It is important that you understand who they are, what specific jobs they do within the clinic, how they share information, and how to reach them when necessary.

To complete the Clinic Contacts Worksheet, review all of the information that you have been given about your clinic, your physicians, and their staff. Also check out their website or, if they use one, a patient portal, which is an online care management site. If the information you need to fill out the Clinic Contacts Worksheet is not readily avail-able, call your clinic and find out if you have been assigned a patient coordinator or head nurse, and ask them who handles things like medical records, scheduling, billing, and insurance issues. Some clinics have dedicated lab or embryology staff that you can add to your contact list, but in many cases lab information will be communicated to you by your RE, nurse, or another contact at your clinic.

Don't be afraid to ask for the specific contacts and the best way to contact them; your clinic and other providers will appreciate that you understand and respect that specific people have specific job functions.

Next, figure out and take notes on how your clinic operates by filling in the Clinic Operations Worksheets. Start by checking to see if your clinic offers any orientation classes, videos, or training seminars about how things work. If so, those classes or vid-eos can help you complete this chapter. Next, figure out what you should do if you have a medical (or other type) of emergency, and determine what requirements there are for starting your cycle, such as pre-cycle viral testing and release paperwork.

Ask about and understand how cycle appointments get scheduled. Some clinics have set start dates for cycles (where a group of patients start cycling on a specific day), but most have rolling or open schedules where you can start a cycle at any time. Similarly, some clinics schedule all your cycle appointments ahead of time, while at others you need to make appointments as you go. No matter what the case, make sure you fully understand the system and that all your appointments are booked ahead of time, if necessary.

Make special note of how monitoring tests and medication instructions work. When it comes to monitoring tests, ask what the procedure is on test day and if there are any time and location options. Remember that your medication type and/or dose can change as a result of your monitoring tests so ask how and when they will notify you about the results of that days testing, including any new or changing medications. Specifically, will they call or email you the same day, or do you need to call them?

Understand ahead of time how your clinic grades (or rates) embryos, as you may need this information to help you make decisions regarding your transfer procedure. Also determine if there are certain criteria that you will need to meet to reach the milestone of embryo cryopreservation. For instance, many clinics will only freeze embryos that are of a certain quality by a specified day (usually day 5).

Following this, ask if they have certain milestones you need to achieve (such as a certain amount of follicles at egg retrieval) to continue with your cycle, or if there are any reasons, medically or otherwise, that your cycle could be canceled. Finally, finish the Clinic Operations Worksheets by asking your contacts at the clinic anything else that is important to you, or whether there is any additional information they think will be helpful to know.

Medications and testing drive an IVF cycle, but are often provided by sources other than your clinic, or at affiliate or "satellite" locations. Upon researching this you may be (pleasantly) surprised to find a testing site or pharmacy that is closer to you, easier to use, or less expensive than previously thought. The Clinic Affiliations Worksheet helps you keep track of satellites and alternative locations as well as companies that you may use in conjunction with your clinic. These can include pharmacies, testing labs, genetic testing and carrier screening companies, couriers (which handle the shipment of lab samples), and more.

The Personal Physicians and Specialists list is important because you may need to access and share their information at a moment's notice. For example, it is not uncommon for a clinic to request general medical or specialist information and documentation, such as a recent physical, PAP, or urology exam, prior to or during a cycle.

This chapter closes with a Clinic Questions Worksheet that you can use to remember things you want to address during your next call or appointment. You can also use it (and the closing Clinic Notes page) to document information you receive during appointments and calls.

When dealing with any provider, always remember that your village is not just working *for* you, they are working *with* you. You are as much a part of the team as anyone, so speak up! This holiest of processes is not to be taken lightly, so make sure you are comfortable with your providers so that you can become a part of the conversation, not just a bystander. Adjusting to this type of multiple practitioner or "village" mentality may feel uncomfortable at first, but doing so is a great way to start a cycle. Things will always be less stressful if you know before you go!

CLINIC CONTACTS WORKSHEET

Clinic: _____

Main Number: _____ Emergency Line: _____

Fax Number: _____ Website: _____

Address: _____ City: _____ State: _____ Zip: _____

Patient Portal/Website: _____

Log In or ID: _____ Password: _____

Reproductive Endocrinologist (RE): _____

Phone: _____ Fax: _____ Email: _____

Patient Coordinator: _____

Phone: _____ Fax: _____ Email: _____

Team Nurse(s): _____

Phone: _____ Fax: _____ Email: _____

Embryologist / Lab Contact: _____

Phone: _____ Fax: _____ Email: _____

Billing: _____

Phone: _____ Fax: _____ Email: _____

Insurance Coordinator: _____

Phone: _____ Fax: _____ Email: _____

Medical Records Contact: _____

Phone: _____ Fax: _____ Email: _____

Other Contact: _____

Phone: _____ Fax: _____ Email: _____

CLINIC OPERATIONS WORKSHEET

Orientation and Training Information:

_____

_____

_____

After-Hours and Emergency Procedure:

_____

_____

_____

Requirements to Start Cycle:

_____

_____

_____

Cycle Start and Appointment Scheduling Information:

_____

_____

_____

Monitoring/Testing Information:

_____

_____

_____

CLINIC OPERATIONS WORKSHEET

Medication Instructions Information:

_____

_____

_____

Embryo Grading Information and Freezing Criteria:

_____

_____

_____

Criteria for Cycle Completion/Possible Causes of Cycle Cancelation:

_____

_____

_____

Additional Information:

_____

_____

_____

Additional Information:

_____

_____

_____

CLINIC AFFILIATIONS WORKSHEET

Clinic Satellite Location: _____

Main Number: _____ Contact: _____

Fax Number: _____ Website/Email: _____

Address: _____ City: _____ State: _____ Zip: _____

Info/Policy/Hours: _____

Pharmacy: _____

Main Number: _____ Contact: _____

Fax Number: _____ Website/Email: _____

Address: _____ City: _____ State: _____ Zip: _____

Info/Policy/Hours: _____

Alternative Pharmacy: _____

Main Number: _____ Contact: _____

Fax Number: _____ Website/Email: _____

Address: _____ City: _____ State: _____ Zip: _____

Info/Policy/Hours: _____

Other: _____

Main Number: _____ Contact: _____

Fax Number: _____ Website/Email: _____

Address: _____ City: _____ State: _____ Zip: _____

Info/Policy/Hours: _____

CLINIC AFFILIATIONS WORKSHEET

Other: _____

Main Number: _____ Contact: _____

Fax Number: _____ Website/Email: _____

Address: _____ City: _____ State: ____ Zip: ____

Info/Policy/Hours: _____

Other: _____

Main Number: _____ Contact: _____

Fax Number: _____ Website/Email: _____

Address: _____ City: _____ State: ____ Zip: ____

Info/Policy/Hours: _____

Other: _____

Main Number: _____ Contact: _____

Fax Number: _____ Website/Email: _____

Address: _____ City: _____ State: ____ Zip: ____

Info/Policy/Hours: _____

Other: _____

Main Number: _____ Contact: _____

Fax Number: _____ Website/Email: _____

Address: _____ City: _____ State: ____ Zip: ____

Info/Policy/Hours: _____

Personal Physician Practice: _____

Main Number: _____ Emergency Line: _____

Fax Number: _____ Website: _____

Address: _____ City: _____ State: _____ Zip: _____

Doctor: _____ Email: _____

OB/GYN Practice: _____

Main Number: _____ Emergency Line: _____

Fax Number: _____ Website: _____

Address: _____ City: _____ State: _____ Zip: _____

Doctor: _____ Email: _____

Urology Practice: _____

Main Number: _____ Emergency Line: _____

Fax Number: _____ Website: _____

Address: _____ City: _____ State: _____ Zip: _____

Doctor: _____ Email: _____

Specialist Practice: _____

Main Number: _____ Emergency Line: _____

Fax Number: _____ Website: _____

Address: _____ City: _____ State: _____ Zip: _____

Doctor: _____ Email: _____

PERSONAL PHYSICIANS AND SPECIALISTS

Other: _____

Main Number: _____ Emergency Line: _____

Fax Number: _____ Website: _____

Address: _____ City: _____ State: _____ Zip: _____

Doctor: _____ Email: _____

Other: _____

Main Number: _____ Emergency Line: _____

Fax Number: _____ Website: _____

Address: _____ City: _____ State: _____ Zip: _____

Doctor: _____ Email: _____

Other: _____

Main Number: _____ Emergency Line: _____

Fax Number: _____ Website: _____

Address: _____ City: _____ State: _____ Zip: _____

Doctor: _____ Email: _____

Other: _____

Main Number: _____ Emergency Line: _____

Fax Number: _____ Website: _____

Address: _____ City: _____ State: _____ Zip: _____

Doctor: _____ Email: _____

CLINIC QUESTIONS WORKSHEET

Appointment or Call Date: _____

Questions: _____

Response/Other Info: _____

_____

Appointment or Call Date: _____

Questions: _____

Response/Other Info: _____

_____

Appointment or Call Date: _____

Questions: _____

Response/Other Info: _____

_____

Appointment or Call Date: _____

Questions: _____

Response/Other Info: _____

_____

Appointment or Call Date: _____

Questions: _____

Response/Other Info: _____

_____

_____

_____

_____

_____

_____

_____

_____

_____

_____

_____

_____

_____

_____

_____

_____

_____

_____

_____

_____

_____

_____

SECTION III
FINANCES

Chapter 5

FINANCES AND IVF:
LAYING THE GROUNDWORK

FOR MANY, DEALING with finances can be boring at best and stressful at worst. But the fact remains that IVF is not cheap, and discussing finances are unfortunately a must when it comes to cycling. Only you (and your partner) can stay on top of the financial aspects of your cycle, and although it might take some work, paying attention to the financial details will keep surprises and aggravation to a minimum while making sure you don't waste time and money.

Before you cycle, you will need to figure out how much things cost, and who, how, and when you will pay for them. Once you have determined those things, it is *your* job to keep track of your expenses and payments, which is particularly important if you are dealing with insurance companies or national healthcare programs, or if you plan on making tax deductions.

Every country in the world has different laws and healthcare systems that govern IVF and other fertility treatments. As a result, costs and coverage levels vary widely depending on *where* you are cycling. Some of the countries that offer some financial assistance, through national or regional healthcare plans, are: Canada, the United States, the United Kingdom, Spain, Australia, Belgium, Denmark, France, Greece, Slovenia, and Sweden. In some cases coverage is complete, but in most there is only partial coverage, and many of these countries have coverage restrictions and waiting lists for covered treatment.

In the United States, coverage mandates vary from state to state, and coverage specifics are usually determined by your employer's insurance program. In Canada, on the other hand, IVF may be covered by Medicare, which is governed by each province's health ministry. In the United Kingdom, coverage is governed by a lottery system run by the National Healthcare System. Restrictions on coverage and the amount of cycles you can receive are based on age and medical condition, as well as by location and whether you've had IVF in the past. In mainland Europe, some countries offer complete coverage, and others only partial coverage; there can also be long waiting lists.

No matter where you are cycling, keeping track of expenses is a necessary evil, and one that has no set standard or practice. Some of the things that can affect the cost of your cycle are:

- Diagnosis and treatment plan
- Clinic and other provider rates and finance plans
- Insurance coverage and healthcare coverage in your state, province, or country

HOW TO USE THIS CHAPTER

Begin figuring out your finances by determining whether you have insurance or healthcare coverage for IVF. If you know that you do not have coverage, go ahead and skip the information and worksheets related to insurance.

FOR PATIENTS WITH INSURANCE COVERAGE

If you are cycling under a non-U.S.-based coverage system, you may need to make adjustments to the worksheets in the insurance section. Use the Finance Notes at the end of the chapter to add information relevant to your situation.

Remember, even if you *have* IVF coverage, most insurance plans and policies have caveats, limits, and maximums, not to mention pages upon pages of fine print, so the number one rule is, *understand your coverage*. The Insurance Coverage Worksheets will get you started, but you also must read your policy, figure out how things like claims processing and referrals work, and stay in contact with your insurance provider.

Start by determining who your provider is and whether you have a member number or some other identification number. Next, figure out how to contact and communicate with them—some insurance providers will have dedicated fertility contacts, and some clinics will have a dedicated staff member or liaison who communicates with your insurance provider on your behalf.

Use the Coverage Details box to review your coverage and determine how many cycles you have covered and what (if any) deductibles and maximum spending caps there are. Next, use the Covered Services box to determine what specific treatments are included. Some providers break up IVF treatment into separate parts, each of which might require a co-payment or have a number or code attached to it that you will need to note.

Next use the Restrictions and Requirements box. Some insurance policies will require that you have certain tests or procedures performed before cycling or that your hormone levels or partner's semen sample meet certain criteria for coverage to be granted. There may also be restrictions to coverage, things that will not be covered such as medications and ancillary items, such as ICSI, certain genetic and other tests, and the cryopreservation of embryos. Some "uncovered services" such as OCPs (oral contraceptive pills), required physicals, or PAP tests may be covered by general insurance, so make sure to check to see if any uncovered services are actually covered by another part of your policy.

In the last box, you can determine who will pay your clinic and other providers such as pharmacies. If the insurance provider does not pay directly, what referral and claims processing procedure will you need to follow to be reimbursed? How and when will that happen? Include information such as referral or identification numbers for your clinic and physicians.

As your treatment progresses, use the Insurance Contact Log to help keep an accurate record of your contact with your provider and any and all claims and reimbursements.

FOR ALL PATIENTS

The majority of patients pay for most or all of their treatment, and even those with insurance coverage usually incur some expenses. No matter what your situation, the best thing you can do is to be prepared by figuring out what your expenses will look like, and how and when you will need to pay them. Use the Cycle Pricing Worksheet and the Payment and Billing Worksheet to do this.

Start by figuring out how your clinic bills for an IVF cycle. Determine if they charge a set price for a cycle or if they charge separately, by item. If they charge a set price, make sure to ask what, if any, procedures or items are not included. For example, at many clinics procedures such as assisted hatching, ICSI, PGD (pre-implantation genetic diagnosis) or other genetic tests are not included in a basic cycle and will incur an additional charge.

Finances and IVF: Laying the Groundwork

Don't assume all of your medications are included in the cost of your cycle. Medicine that is given to you at the clinic, such as anesthesia, *may* be included, but most of the time the bulk of cycle medications such as OCPs, stimulation and suppression medications, and progesterone or estrogen support will be acquired and paid for separately, outside of your clinic.

To figure out your Total Cycle Expenses on the Cycle Pricing Worksheet, review and complete each expense category by filling in the quoted price for each item or by filling in the amount of a set price cycle and checking the box next to items that are included in that set price. There is also a section for miscellaneous expenses, which includes items that are not necessarily part of your cycle, but that many patients spend money on. It is a good idea to include these types of expenses so that you will have a realistic picture of *all* your expenses, not just the ones related to your clinic. When you are done, use the Total Cycle Expenses box to add everything up.

Once you know how much you will be spending you can review your options for financing and payment plans. Many clinics and private companies offer financing and shared risk or refund programs, which allow patients to save money on multiple cycles, or to get a partial refund if a pregnancy is not achieved. These programs can be a great way to save money but *do* require research and may have acceptance restrictions, so make sure to read the fine print and consult with your clinic about the best options for you. Use the Payment Options box to document the options available to you.

Once you determine how you will pay for your treatment, use the Payment Information box to determine payment methods, billing schedules, and any requirements for payment, such as due dates and method of payment. You can use the master calendar in Chapter 7 to log any payment due dates you need to remember.

As your cycle progresses, keep track of expenses and payments by using the Payment Tracking Log. This log will become extremely valuable if you plan on making tax deductions, which will be covered in the next chapter. To use the log, simply note the vendor (whom you paid), invoice number (if you have one), and the amount due. When you make a payment you can fill in the amount and type. Remember to make sure you save your receipts—you may need them!

Keeping a clear record of payments ensures that you will have all the necessary information at your fingertips if a question regarding payment arises, and can help you easily determine and document any upcoming expenses.

INSURANCE COVERAGE WORKSHEET

Insurance Provider Information

Company or Agency: _____ Member ID # _____

Main Number: _____ Emergency Line: _____

Address: _____ City: _____ State: _____ Zip: _____

Fax Number: _____ Website: _____

Web Login ID: _____ Web Password: _____

Infertility Contact Line: _____ Contact Name: _____

IVF Clinic Insurance Liaison: _____ Phone: _____

Coverage Details:

Coverage Overview/Number of Cycles Included: _____

_____

_____

Annual Deductible: _____ Annual Max Spend: _____

Lifetime Max Spend: _____

Covered Services

Service: _____ Co-Pay Amount: _____

Ins. Code / Other Info: _____

Service: _____ Co-Pay Amount: _____

Ins. Code / Other Info: _____

Service: _____ Co-Pay Amount: _____

Ins. Code / Other Info: _____

Service: _____ Co-Pay Amount: _____

Ins. Code / Other Info: _____

INSURANCE COVERAGE WORKSHEET

Restrictions and Requirements

Requirements for IVF Coverage: _____

_____

_____

Services Not Covered:

_____   _____

_____   _____

_____   _____

_____   _____

_____   _____

_____   _____

_____   _____

Payments, Referrals, Claims and Reimbursements

Clinic Paid by Insurance Provider or Patient: _____

Payment/Claims Processing Procedure and Timing: _____

_____

_____

_____

Referrals Procedure: _____

_____

Reproductive Endocrinologist Referral I.D. _____

Primary Physician Referral I.D. _____

INSURANCE CONTACT LOG

Date/Time: _____ Spoke to: _____ Confirmation #: _____

Reason/Results/Follow-Up: _____

_____

_____

Date/Time: _____ Spoke to: _____ Confirmation #: _____

Reason/Results/Follow-Up: _____

_____

_____

Date/Time: _____ Spoke to: _____ Confirmation #: _____

Reason/Results/Follow-Up: _____

_____

_____

Date/Time: _____ Spoke to: _____ Confirmation #: _____

Reason/Results/Follow-Up: _____

_____

_____

Date/Time: _____ Spoke to: _____ Confirmation #: _____

Reason/Results/Follow-Up: _____

_____

_____

CYCLE PRICING WORKSHEET

Set Price For Cycle? No / Yes   If Yes, Amount For One Cycle $_____

Administrative Expenses
Administrative Fee/Consult $_____
Lab Fees $_____
Office Visits $_____
Storage Fees $_____
Other _____ $_____
Total Admin Expenses $_____

Testing Expenses
Day Three Testing $_____
Carrier Screening $_____
Genetic Testing $_____
Monitoring, Bloodwork $_____
Monitoring, Ultrasound $_____
Pregnancy Monitoring $_____
Pregnancy Test $_____
Semen Analysis $_____
Viral / Infectious Disease $_____
Other _____ $_____
Total Testing Expenses $_____

Medication Expenses
Anesthesia $_____
Antibiotic $_____
Injections $_____
Oral $_____
Patch $_____
Other _____ $_____
Total Medication Expenses $_____

Procedural Expenses
Assisted Hatching $_____
Egg Retrieval $_____
Embryo Cryopreservation $_____
Embryo Storage $_____
Embryo Transfer $_____
Embryo Screening $_____
ICSI $_____
Sperm Cryopreservation $_____
Sperm Washing $_____
Other _____ $_____
Total Procedural Expenses $_____

Misc. Expenses
Acupuncture $_____
Courier Fees $_____
Gas/Tolls $_____
Hotel/Lodging $_____
Home Pregnancy Tests $_____
Legal/Agency Fees $_____
Therapy $_____
Yoga $_____
Other _____ $_____
Other _____ $_____
Other _____ $_____
Total Misc. Expenses $_____

Total Cycle Expenses
Clinic Set Price $_____
Total Admin Expenses $_____
Total Testing Expenses $_____
Total Medication Expenses $_____
Total Procedural Expenses $_____
Total Misc. Expenses $_____
Total Cycle Expenses $_____

PAYMENT AND BILLING WORKSHEET

Payment Options:

Payment Plans Available: _____

_____

_____

Multi-Cycle Packages/Shared Risk/Refund Program Information: _____

_____

_____

_____

Payment Information:

Selected Plan (If Any): _____

_____

Payment Schedule: _____

_____

_____

_____

_____

Billing Requirements: _____

_____

_____

_____

_____

_____

Vendor	Date	Invoice #	Amount Due	Amount Paid	Payment Type

_____

_____

_____

_____

_____

_____

_____

_____

_____

_____

_____

_____

_____

_____

_____

_____

_____

_____

_____

_____

_____

Chapter 6

IVF AND TAXES:
A GUIDE FOR US CITIZENS

FERTILITY TREATMENTS, INCLUDING IVF procedures, surgeries, ultrasounds, medicines, and even pregnancy tests may be tax deductible, but when tax time actually rolls around, many of us ignore the possibility of deducting fertility expenses. Some of us dread it; some of us fear it; most of us don't completely understand it; but, because you may have a shot at getting some of your hard-earned money back, it is absolutely worth looking into.

As of 2013, the IRS rule is that you can deduct only the amount of your medical expenses that is more than 7.5% of your Adjusted Gross Income (AGI). Sound confusing? That's because it is; but if you have kept records of your medical spending, and take things step by step, you can figure out in no time whether your IVF and other medical expenses can be deducted on your tax return and how to do it.

If you have an accountant, by all means let them handle things, but for the general population who prepare taxes on their own, you must first figure out if you qualify for deductions and, if so, how much you can deduct. Here are the steps to take:

STEP ONE: READ THE RULES. As if medical deductions weren't complicated enough, the IRS has a lot of rules, restrictions, and guidelines regarding what expenses, income levels, persons, and situations qualify for medical deductions. The good news is that they spell these rules out clearly each year in IRS Publication 502 "Medical and Dental Expenses." This publication, which is frequently updated by the IRS, offers detailed information on what expenses, income levels, persons, and situations qualify for medical deductions. This information can be found at www.irs.gov/publications.

STEP TWO: ADD IT UP. Add up all of your qualified medical expenses for the year. Remember that you can include *all* of your medical expenses, not just those related to fertility treatment. If you have been keeping track of expenses and saving bills and receipts, you are ahead of the game. If not, be ready to roll up your sleeves and dig a bit. If you didn't save records, you will have to rely on bank statements and canceled checks. If necessary, you can ask your providers to provide receipts after the fact.

STEP THREE: DETERMINE YOUR INCOME. Your Adjusted Gross Income (AGI) is your total income from taxable sources, minus allowable deductions such as student loan interest, education expenses, contributions to an IRA, or contributions to a health savings or flexible spending accounts. You must complete your main tax form 1040 to figure out your AGI. Only then can you determine if you're eligible to make medical expense deductions.

STEP FOUR: DO THE MATH. Once you know your total medical expenses and your AGI you can use the Tax Planner in this chapter to do the math which is relatively straightforward (though for most of us, a calculator helps!).

The Worksheets in this chapter will walk you through the above steps; but, like infertility treatment, deducting medical expenses can be confusing, and is always unique to each person's situation. It also takes a good amount of time, so the help of a professional is the best way to go! If you go it alone, here are a few more things to keep in mind:

- You *must* have documentation, such as receipts, mileage logs, and medical records to back up any deductions you make. Refer to www.IRS.gov or your accountant to help you determine what qualifies as appropriate documentation.

- Tax law and IRS publications are updated every year and are subject to change, so make sure you have the latest information when preparing taxes.

- Deducting medical expenses is not as straightforward as it may seem and IRS guidelines can be complicated. You can only deduct certain expenses and amounts in certain situations. For example, if you travel for your IVF treatment, you may be able to deduct the cost of lodging if all of the following requirements are met*:

---

* *Qualification guidelines based on the 2012 IRS Publication 502 "Medical and Dental Expenses."*

1. The lodging is primarily for, and essential to, medical care.

2. The medical care is provided by a doctor in a licensed hospital or in a medical care facility related to, or the equivalent of, a licensed hospital.

3. The lodging is not lavish or extravagant under the circumstances.

4. There is no significant element of personal pleasure, recreation, or vacation in the travel away from home.

5. The amount you include in medical expenses for lodging cannot be more than $50 for each night for each person. You can include lodging for a person traveling with the person receiving the medical care.

HOW TO USE THIS CHAPTER

Start by figuring out how much money you spent on IVF and infertility-related medical expenses by completing the IVF Expenses Worksheet. If you used the Cycle Pricing Worksheet and the Payment Tracking Log from Chapter 5 you are well on your way. If not, you will need to refer to old bills, receipts, canceled checks, credit card statements, and so on.

Remember that the IVF Expenses Worksheet list only covers items commonly related to IVF and infertility treatment—if you have other medical expenses not listed on the IVF Expenses Worksheet or not related to IVF and infertility you will need to determine if those are deductible as well. IRS Publication 502, "Medical and Dental Expenses," can help you determine all possible qualifying medical expenses.

Use the first box on the IVF Tax Planner Worksheet to figure out your total medical expenses by adding the amount of your IVF and infertility expenses to the amount of all your other qualifying medical expenses.

Once you know your total medical expenses you can use the next two boxes to determine if you qualify for deductions, and if so, calculate how much you can deduct. The Tax Planner Worksheet will walk you through these steps.

Remember, taxes are complicated, and even if you think you qualify, professional advice is still very helpful!

IVF EXPENSES WORKSHEET

Only certain expenses qualify for tax deductions. The list provided here is a partial list of items commonly related to IVF and infertility. For a complete list see IRS Publication 502 "Medical and Dental Expenses" at www.irs.gov/publications.

IRS Deductible Category	Total Spent
Acupuncture	$_____
Bandages (Medical Supplies)	$_____
Birth Control Pills	$_____
Body Scan (Ultrasound)	$_____
Fertility Enhancement (Procedures and Surgeries)	$_____
Health Institute	$_____
Health Maintenance Organization (HMO)	$_____
Hospital Services	$_____
Laboratory Fees	$_____
Lodging	$_____
Meals	$_____
Medical Conferences	$_____
Medicines	$_____
Operations	$_____
Physical Examination	$_____
Pregnancy Test Kit	$_____
Psychoanalysis	$_____
Psychologist	$_____
Therapy	$_____
Transportation	$_____
Trips	$_____

Total IVF and Infertility-Related Expenses: $_____

TAX PLANNER WORKSHEET

Figuring Out Your Total Medical Expenses

IVF and Infertility-Related Expenses: $_____
                       +
Other Qualified Medical Expenses: $_____
                       =
     Total Medical Expenses: $_____

Determining If You Qualify for Deductions

You can deduct the amount of your medical expenses that is more than 7.5% of your Adjusted Gross Income (AGI). AGI is your total income from taxable sources minus allowable deductions and can be found on form 1040 on your tax return.

For example, if your AGI is $40,000 then 7.5% of that income (your qualifying amount) is $3,000.00.

    Adjusted Gross Income: $_____
    x
    7.5%
    =
    $_____ is 7.5% of your AGI. This is your Qualifying Amount.

To make deductions, your Total Medical Expenses must be larger than your Qualifying Amount.

Total Medical Expenses: $_____   Qualifying Amount: $_____

If your Qualifying Amount is larger than your Total Medical Expenses you cannot make a deduction.

Calculating the Amount You Can Deduct If You Qualify

If your Total Medical Expenses are more than your Qualifying Amount you can deduct the difference. For example if you paid medical expenses of $3,500.00 and your Qualifying Amount is $3,000.00 then you can deduct $500.00.

        Total Medical Expenses $_____
                   -
        Qualifying Amount $_____
                   =
                $_____ is the amount you can deduct.

Section IV
IVF Cycle

Chapter 7

CYCLE SCHEDULE, YOUR LIFE: UNDER CONSTRUCTION

I LIKE TO THINK of an IVF cycle as being like a construction zone. The yellow lights are flashing, lanes are shifting, and there is heavy equipment in the area. It is time to slow down, read the signs, and be a bit more cautious than usual. In order to do this, you must listen to your mind and body and take it easy. For many of us "taking it easy" is very hard (if not impossible) to accomplish. But when undergoing IVF it is crucial, and can be as simple as this: just don't do everything you normally do.

If this seems impossible, try acknowledging that your cycle is a set period of time. It may feel like an eternity to you and your partner, but in the grand scheme of things a cycle doesn't last very long—six to eight weeks tops, and then you are done. As you begin to work your cycle into your regular schedule and progress through this period of time, here are a few suggestions on how you can actually slow down and take it easy during a cycle:

- Don't commit to unnecessary social engagements. Click the "maybe" button as much as you can. That way if you *are* feeling up to it you can go, but if you are not, you will have an easy out.

- Avoid new, high-stress projects and be careful not to overschedule yourself. Review deadlines and events ahead of time, and leave plenty of extra time to finish projects.

- Plan time to rest. Even if you don't end up needing it, is comforting to know you have the option to check out for a few minutes (or hours) if you feel like it.

- If you are cycling during a holiday or large social event, consider opting for convenience, even if it is not your norm. There is always next year for perfect gifts, complicated recipes, and lavish decorations.

- If you are finding it difficult, consider setting limits on child-focused activities. If you feel committed, remember that it is perfectly acceptable to just "stop by" at baby showers and birthday parties to drop off a gift or give a quick hello. You can also offer to help with set-up or clean-up in an effort to avoid the actual event.

It may seem unnecessary now, but taking concrete steps to free up your schedule during your cycle will leave you with more mental and physical energy later on, should you need it. Remember that this is not a permanent situation. Before you know it, the "End Work Zone" sign will appear and you will be back up to speed.

HOW TO COMPLETE THIS CHAPTER

This chapter focuses on the schedule and timing of your IVF cycle. Before you begin, consider reviewing your Treatment Worksheet on page 29, the Clinic Operations Worksheet on pages 38–39, and the IVF Basics section so you can be as familiar as possible with the process as you plan your cycle.

As you complete this chapter keep in mind that all of your dates are subject to change. My advice: use a pencil! Things can change quickly and often during a cycle, so you may need to make adjustments.

Start the Cycle Schedule Worksheet by listing what event will mark your cycle start date. Your start date will be dictated by your treatment plan and may be based on the first day of your period, your baseline ultrasound (also referred to as a suppression check), or some other milestone, such as beginning oral contraceptives or another medication.

Next, fill in the Estimated Date column by using information provided by your clinic. The items listed on this worksheet follow a basic cycle schedule, and the actual process may flow a bit differently for some patients. For example, not all cycles require OCPs, and the number of monitoring tests is not always five—it can be more or less.

You can fill in the Actual Date Column when you learn your exact dates, which can be as late as the day before the event itself. If your clinic calendar includes details and instructions about cycle events you can document them on the Cycle Schedule Notes page.

After you have completed the Cycle Schedule Worksheet you can fill in the Calendar Pages. This will be your master calendar, as it provides a three-month overview with enough space to include pre-cycle events, as well as the waiting period after your transfer. The calendar can be used for appointments, tests, results, instructions, complementary treatments, budgetary reminders, and non-cycle commitments that coincide with or may affect cycle events.

Begin by filling in the corresponding month at the top of the page. Because IVF cycles are usually run by numbered cycle days, two boxes are provided for each day so you can enter both the day number (calendar date) and cycle day (usually provided by your clinic).

As you work on your schedule remember that, like all things related to IVF, dates, times, and events are always subject to change!

CYCLE SCHEDULE WORKSHEET

Cycle Start Date Based On: _____

	Estimated Date/Cycle Day	Actual Date/Cycle Day
Cycle Start:		
OCP Start:		
Suppression Medication Start:		
Baseline Ultrasound (Suppression Check):		
Stimulation Medication Start:		
Monitoring Tests:		
Monitoring Tests:		
Monitoring Tests:		
Monitoring Tests:		
Monitoring Tests:		
HCG Trigger:		
Egg Retrieval:		
Progesterone Medication Start:		
Embryo Transfer:		
Pregnancy Test:		
Other: _____		

_____

_____

_____

_____

_____

_____

_____

_____

_____

_____

_____

_____

_____

_____

_____

_____

_____

_____

_____

_____

CYCLE SCHEDULE NOTES

MONTH _____

MONTH

Chapter 8

A Spoonful of Sugar: Medications, Stimulation and Procedures

Y OU MAY ALREADY be taking some medications, and have had quite a few appointments, but during the stimulation and the procedural phases of your cycle there is, to put it lightly, a *lot* going on!

When you reach this point you may find yourself overwhelmed by the amount of time and attention required. During stimulation you will likely be taking multiple medicines, going to frequent monitoring appointments, receiving daily instructions and, of course, mentally gearing up for the big procedures: egg retrieval and embryo transfer. As the physical, hormonal and emotional pressures combine with your everyday obligations, it can be hard to stay positive and not lose yourself in the daily details of cycling.

Of course, a 6 a.m. blood draw and trans-vaginal ultrasound are not high on anyone's list of fun things to do, but if you can associate these and other obligatory cycle events with a positive feeling or experience you can minimize the stress and tension that they create. You can do this by using rituals, which are a great way to add some positive energy and help to remember to take care of yourself while you cycle.

For example, when you get up an extra hour (or two!) early to make it to monitoring before work, let yourself have that special (sigh, decaf) coffee drink; you know, the one that has too many calories and costs a few extra bucks. If coffee's not your thing, try a fat glossy magazine to read in the waiting room or some new music or apps for your phone to keep you busy. You don't have to break the bank, but if a little indulgence is going to make your experience more pleasant, it is worth it in the long run. When it comes to those pesky injections, try rewarding yourself after you administer each shot. A Hershey kiss or a little massage from your partner is a great way to associate shots with something comforting. You probably will never look forward to the shot, but if you are consistent, you can look past the shot and forward to the little treat.

Retrieval and transfer days are a great time to come home with your favorite takeout and a movie, or to plan on watching that marathon of Top Model you have stashed on your DVR. Get a post-retrieval pedicure (as you'll be staring at your toes for a while during transfer) or book a massage for the afternoon after your transfer. Let your partner pamper you by preparing dinner so you can stay relaxed on the couch. If you know you will be on bed rest after transfer, prepare ahead of time by setting out books, magazines, your iPod, computer, your journal, or whatever it is you like, so you can actually enjoy the downtime.

In short, if you think of all your cycle responsibilities as chores or as negative events to be survived, your cycle will be pretty hard to get through. Attaching positive rituals and events to the process is an excellent way to make a cycle survivable and a sweeter way to help the medicine go down, so to speak.

HOW TO USE SECTION ONE OF THIS CHAPTER

This chapter is broken into two sections. The first section focuses on medicines and stimulation, including hormone levels and follicle growth. The second section will cover procedures and embryos.

The Medication Details Worksheet will prompt you to list the different types of medications you will be taking, what form they come in (pill, injection, patch, etc.) and their individual usage and storage instructions (do they need to be refrigerated, etc.). As you complete the worksheet, it is a good idea to save all complicated prescription instructions, including those for injections; keep them in a dedicated place, as you may need to reference them when administering medications. Some pharmacies and drug makers provide USBs (also known as thumb drives) with pre-loaded instructions, while others offer online video instruction and phone support, so you may want to make a note of that information as well.

The Medication Log will help you to keep track of the medications you will be taking throughout your cycle. I recommend using your cycle start date as the first day of the log and filling in the dates and cycle days first. Once you have done that you can fill in the name of the medications you will be taking, starting with the first (usually OCPs or suppression medications) and ending with the last (usually progesterone). Keep in mind that not all patients will need to use all five rows all the time. At some points in your cycle you will only be taking one or two different medications; at others you may take more.

If you know the exact dose, time, and amount of your medications (as is usually the case with OCPs and pre-cycle suppression medications) you can fill them in ahead of time; but in many cases, such as with stimulation medications and the trigger shot, you will need to wait for instructions, including date, time, and dose.

If you fill in the log ahead of time and feel you might have trouble remembering if you took a certain dose, make a check mark or X in the appropriate box when you actually take the medication.

The Stimulation Monitoring and Hormone Level Worksheets that follow allow you to keep track of and view your physical responses to medications and treatment.

The Stimulation Monitoring Worksheet contains three small charts. The first gives an overview of your stimulation activity; the charts that follow track your follicle development on each ovary in more detail. To complete the first chart, fill in the cycle day and date that you receive your monitoring tests and make a check mark in the box for each type of test you have that day (usually blood work and ultrasound). If you have another type of test, you can use the Other column. When you receive the results from your tests, usually toward the end of the day, you can fill in the columns for Total Follicles, Uterine Lining, Estradiol (estrogen), and any other results.

If you wish, you can use the individual ovary charts to note the size and location of your follicles. Some clinics do not readily provide this information, but if you want to know, you can always ask.

The Hormone Levels Worksheet allows you to document your hormone levels. You can elect to use this worksheet only during your stimulation phase, or you can use it to chart your levels throughout your treatment. The worksheet includes four commonly tested hormones, but because different patients are tested for different things, there are also four extra blank charts for you to customize to reflect any additional testing you may be receiving.

MEDICATIONS DETAILS WORKSHEET

Medication: Form: Storage Guidelines:

Instructions For Use:

Medication: Form: Storage Guidelines:

Instructions For Use:

Medication: Form: Storage Guidelines:

Instructions For Use:

Medication: Form: Storage Guidelines:

Instructions For Use:

Medication: Form: Storage Guidelines:

Instructions For Use:

Medication: Form: Storage Guidelines:

Instructions For Use:

Medication: Form: Storage Guidelines:

Instructions For Use:

MEDICATION LOG

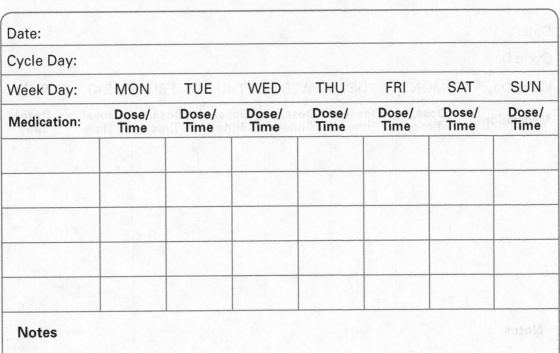

Date:							
Cycle Day:							
Week Day:	MON	TUE	WED	THU	FRI	SAT	SUN
Medication:	Dose/ Time	Dose/ Time	Dose/ Time	Dose/ Time	Dose/ Time	Dose/ Time	Dose/ Time
Notes							

Date:							
Cycle Day:							
Week Day:	MON	TUE	WED	THU	FRI	SAT	SUN
Medication:	Dose/ Time	Dose/ Time	Dose/ Time	Dose/ Time	Dose/ Time	Dose/ Time	Dose/ Time
Notes							

Date:							
Cycle Day:							
Week Day:	MON	TUE	WED	THU	FRI	SAT	SUN
Medication:	Dose/Time	Dose/Time	Dose/Time	Dose/Time	Dose/Time	Dose/Time	Dose/Time
Notes							

Date:							
Cycle Day:							
Week Day:	MON	TUE	WED	THU	FRI	SAT	SUN
Medication:	Dose/Time	Dose/Time	Dose/Time	Dose/Time	Dose/Time	Dose/Time	Dose/Time
Notes							

Date:

Cycle Day:

Week Day:	MON	TUE	WED	THU	FRI	SAT	SUN
Medication:	Dose/ Time	Dose/ Time	Dose/ Time	Dose/ Time	Dose/ Time	Dose/ Time	Dose/ Time

Notes

Date:

Cycle Day:

Week Day:	MON	TUE	WED	THU	FRI	SAT	SUN
Medication:	Dose/ Time	Dose/ Time	Dose/ Time	Dose/ Time	Dose/ Time	Dose/ Time	Dose/ Time

Notes

MEDICATION LOG

Date:

Cycle Day:

Week Day:	MON		TUE		WED		THU		FRI		SAT		SUN	
Medication:	Dose/ Time		Dose/ Time		Dose/ Time		Dose/ Time		Dose/ Time		Dose/ Time		Dose/ Time	

Notes

Date:

Cycle Day:

Week Day:	MON		TUE		WED		THU		FRI		SAT		SUN	
Medication:	Dose/ Time		Dose/ Time		Dose/ Time		Dose/ Time		Dose/ Time		Dose/ Time		Dose/ Time	

Notes

MEDICATION LOG

Date: _____

Cycle Day: _____

Week Day:	MON	TUE	WED	THU	FRI	SAT	SUN
Medication:	Dose/ Time	Dose/ Time	Dose/ Time	Dose/ Time	Dose/ Time	Dose/ Time	Dose/ Time

Notes

Date: _____

Cycle Day: _____

Week Day:	MON	TUE	WED	THU	FRI	SAT	SUN
Medication:	Dose/ Time	Dose/ Time	Dose/ Time	Dose/ Time	Dose/ Time	Dose/ Time	Dose/ Time

Notes

MEDICATION LOG

Date:							
Cycle Day:							
Week Day:	MON	TUE	WED	THU	FRI	SAT	SUN
Medication:	Dose/ Time	Dose/ Time	Dose/ Time	Dose/ Time	Dose/ Time	Dose/ Time	Dose/ Time
Notes							

Date:							
Cycle Day:							
Week Day:	MON	TUE	WED	THU	FRI	SAT	SUN
Medication:	Dose/ Time	Dose/ Time	Dose/ Time	Dose/ Time	Dose/ Time	Dose/ Time	Dose/ Time
Notes							

STIMULATION MONITORING WORKSHEET

Stimulation Monitoring Overview

Date	Cycle Day	Ultra Sound	Blood Work	Total Follicles	Uterine Lining	Estradiol	Other	Other	Other

Right Ovary

Date	Cycle Day	Total Follicles	Sizes/Range

Left Ovary

Date	Cycle Day	Total Follicles	Sizes/Range

HORMONE LEVELS WORKSHEET

Estradiol	
Date	**Level**

Progesterone	
Date	**Level**

LH	
Date	**Level**

FSH	
Date	**Level**

Date	**Level**

Date	**Level**

Date	**Level**

Date	**Level**

HOW TO USE SECTION TWO
OF THIS CHAPTER

The next section in this chapter covers the procedural elements of your cycle, including egg retrieval, fertilization, and embryo growth, and transfer. If you are not familiar with this phase of treatment, you may want to review the IVF Basics section (page 9) before you get started.

Start with the Egg Retrieval Planning Worksheet which begins with space where you can fill in the details of your trigger (HCG) shot and your egg retrieval. Remember that this information will not be set in stone until the end of your stimulation phase.

However, even without having the exact date, you can still make sure you have all the necessary information, including the time and location of your egg retrieval procedure; any specific instructions for that day; information about what you can (and cannot) eat prior; as well as what to wear, what to bring, and what you can expect from the procedure. Make sure to include any instructions for your partner regarding on-site semen samples, or transferring pre-collected or frozen samples.

If you are nervous about the procedure take some time to ask your nurse or MD to review the process with you and make a Retrieval Day Plan to ease your mind. Share your plan with your partner or the person who will be accompanying you that day, and include travel and timing logistics and any other information such as directions to the site, coverage for work, pets and other errands. You may not receive post-retrieval instructions until after the procedure, but feel free to ask ahead of time if you would like to know in advance.

Once the procedure is complete you will learn your results and can fill in the Egg Retrieval Results Worksheet which includes how many follicles were present, how many eggs were retrieved and how many were mature. It also includes a section for information on your partner's semen sample. Semen sample information may not be available immediately after the procedure but you can ask for a report after the procedure to complete the semen sample information section of the worksheet.

The Fertilization and Embryo Growth Worksheet covers the time in between your retrieval and transfer which is usually 3 or 5 days. You will be able to fill out the Initial Fertilization Call box when you receive notification regarding how many eggs have fertilized, usually in the form of a call or email the day after your retrieval.

You can use the Embryo Growth Information box to record information about your growing embryos. To use the box note the date, cycle day and how many embryos you have. In the section for size and description you can record more detailed information, such as the number of cells making up each embryo or their current grade or rating. Keep in mind that while some clinics automatically provide a daily update on embryo growth, many do not so if you want this type of information you may have to ask for it specifically.

Many patients are surprised to find that the time between egg retrieval and transfer can be quite stressful as you wait to hear about your developing embryos. There is also a chance that some patients may hit bumps in the road during this phase. If you find this time difficult, don't hesitate to use the advice in Section V: Wait and Results, and Section VI: Support for Mind and Body to get you through this period.

During this time, based on your developing embryos, it will be determined whether your planned transfer day will stay the same or change. Once you know the exact date of your transfer, you can make specific plans for that day; however, it is a good idea to have a general idea of what to expect beforehand. Use the Embryo Transfer Worksheet to help you understand the basic details of your transfer and what pre- and post- instructions look like.

After your transfer you can fill in the details about the number and grade (or type) of embryos that were transferred. You can also note any additional procedures such as assisted hatching or any genetic testing such as PGD or CGH. If you have extra embryos left to freeze, you can note that here as well. Keep in mind that many clinics do not automatically tell you how many embryos were frozen, so you may have to call and ask or wait to receive information in the mail. Also, most clinics have specific criteria for freezing embryos, such as their being a certain size, or their grade on Day 5 so you may want to review your Clinic Operations Worksheets on these subjects prior to transfer.

As you complete this phase of your cycle just remember that although the road you are traveling might be bumpy, and might even have become a bit re-arranged since you first started, it is still basically the same road. Just slow down a bit and pay attention to the signs that your body, heart and mind are giving you, and you'll get out of the construction zone before you know it, safe and sound.

EGG RETRIEVAL PLANNING WORKSHEET

Trigger (HCG) Shot Information:

Date: _____ Cycle Day: _____ Exact Time: _____

Dose & Instruction: _____

Egg Retrieval Information:

Date: _____ Cycle Day: _____ Arrival Time: _____

Location: _____

Retrieval Day Instructions:

_____

_____

Semen Sample Instructions:

_____

_____

Retrieval Day Plan:

_____

_____

Post-Retrieval Instructions:

_____

_____

EGG RETRIEVAL RESULTS WORKSHEET

Egg Retrieval Report

Final Number of Follicles: _____   Eggs Retrieved: _____   Eggs Mature: _____

Notes: _____

_____

_____

_____

_____

_____

Semen Sample Information

Semen Analysis Initial:

Count/Volume: _____   Motility/Forward Progression: _____

Concentration: _____   Morphology/Abnormal Count: _____

Other: _____   Other: _____

Semen Analysis Final (after washing or thaw):

Count/Volume: _____   Motility/Forward Progression: _____

Concentration: _____   Morphology/Abnormal Count: _____

Other: _____   Other: _____

Notes: _____

_____

_____

FERTILIZATION & EMBRYO GROWTH WORKSHEET

Initial Fertilization Call

Number of Eggs Fertilized: _____   Number w/ICSI: _____

Embryo Growth Information

Date: _____   Cycle Day: _____   # of Embryos: _____

Size / Description: _____

_____

_____

Date: _____   Cycle Day: _____   # of Embryos: _____

Size / Description: _____

_____

_____

Date: _____   Cycle Day: _____   # of Embryos: _____

Size / Description: _____

_____

_____

Date: _____   Cycle Day: _____   # of Embryos: _____

Size / Description: _____

_____

_____

Date: _____   Cycle Day: _____   # of Embryos: _____

Size / Description: _____

_____

_____

EMBRYO TRANSFER WORKSHEET

Transfer Information

_____ 3 Day Transfer   _____ 5 Day transfer   _____ Other

Date: _____   Cycle Day: _____   Arrival Time: _____

Location: _____

_____

Transfer Day Instructions and Plan: _____

_____

Post Transfer Instructions: _____

_____

Transfer Results

Number of Embryos Available: _____

Number of Embryos Transferred: _____

Embryo #1   Description / Grade: _____   AH: Y / N

Genetic testing: Y / N_____   Type: _____

Embryo #2   Description / Grade: _____   AH: Y / N

Genetic testing: Y / N_____   Type: _____

Embryo #3   Description / Grade: _____   AH: Y / N

Genetic testing: Y / N_____   Type: _____

Embryo #4   Description / Grade: _____   AH: Y / N

Genetic testing: Y / N_____   Type: _____

Cryopreservation Information

Number of Embryos Frozen: _____   Frozen on Day: _____

SECTION V
WAIT AND
RESULTS

Chapter 9

THE TWO WEEK WAIT & CHANNELING YOUR INNER BEE

WELCOME TO THE "Two-Week Wait": That time between your transfer and your pregnancy test famous for being a slow-moving torture. Grab a seat, kick off your shoes and get comfy; you'll be here for a bit!

While most IVF patients have already experienced a few Two-Week Waits during their infertility career, this one may feel slightly different. Combine the physical rigors of cycling (and getting up at all hours for the past few weeks) with the hangover from the hormonal cocktail that is IVF, and you may find yourself pretty exhausted. It also doesn't help that after the relatively rapid fire pace of stimulation through transfer comes to a close, IVF cycles by nature, go from a flurry of activity to an abrupt halt. There are no more daily calls with the clinic; no more monitoring appointments or procedures; just two long weeks of nothing but progesterone to look forward to. This vacuum can make an IVF Two-Week Wait feel like an eternity and can put you in a position where you need to emotionally readjust, *again*.

For most IVF patients the Two-Week Wait is actually only 9 to 12 days, but no matter how long yours is, having a survival strategy is crucial to staying sane. My advice is to stay busy—very busy.

And yes, it *is* possible to do this, even when you have zero energy from the medications, and you think about your impending results every three to five seconds. Again, it *is* possible; but in order to actually do it, you must make a realistic plan and stick to it. This is not the time to try and engage in new activities, events, or projects that you don't enjoy. Whenever possible, avoid unpleasant events and tasks, but also try to avoid doing nothing (unless of course nothing is your favorite thing), or time will drag and the wait can feel even longer.

At a loss for ideas? The Two-Week Wait Project Planner offers some suggestions. Here are a few of my favorites, but remember: this is not about me, and for this to really work you need to do things that *you* like:

- Plan your next holiday gathering. Plan menus, buy gifts, make travel arrangements, or purchase and write out birthday cards for the next 6 months. This way, whether you find yourself pregnant or dealing with cycling again you will have crossed off some major errands.

- Clean out your closets; clichéd, perhaps, but it works. Closets, drawers, cabinets, basements, attics . . . anything that allows you to get lost in purging, categorizing, and organizing while also enabling you to feel satisfaction at a job well done can't hurt. Just keep in mind that many clinics advise against vigorous activity during the Two-Week Wait, so make sure you are not doing any heavy lifting while you clean.

- If you haven't read Chapter 10 already, do so. Review your clinic's policies about pregnancy testing, notification, and post-cycle treatment, and prep for your results.

- If you can afford a vacation (and have the time off) the Two-Week Wait is an excellent time to take or plan a trip. If money and time are tight, try becoming a tourist for a day. Grab your partner or a friend and go on a local road trip that won't break the bank.

- If you are on bed rest, you will have to get more creative, as there are only so many magazines, movies, and nail polish changes a girl can stomach. Try learning a new language or technology (do you Skype, yet?) or enlist the help of your partner and a few close friends who can spend some time entertaining you (bed party, anyone?). Maybe try writing a blog, where you can vent away about the injustice of infertility, IVF, and bed rest. Finally, if all else fails, remember all those mornings when you would have given anything for a few more minutes of shut eye, and try to enjoy the downtime.

HOW TO USE THIS CHAPTER

The chapter begins with a Two-Week Wait Project Planner, which encourages you to plan activities that are based on your possible moods (which, as I've mentioned, can change quickly and often). You should also include activities of varying lengths so you will always have a go-to activity whether you need to fill 10 minutes, a few hours, or a whole day.

You can use the Two-Week Wait Calendar to fill in the days of your wait with Project Planner activities and any other activities that you will engage in for each specific day. Ideally, you should make these plans *before* the Two-Week Wait, but the planning can be an activity in itself. One way or another, you should try to fill in as many possible activities as you can, and revisit this calendar when time is seemingly grinding to a halt.

The Two-Week Wait Observation Log provides a venue for tracking physical and emotional observations during the Two-Week Wait, and can be used in many different ways, as you see fit.

For instance, during the Two-Week Wait you may find that you can't stop obsessing over possible pregnancy symptoms. This can be very frustrating because at any given minute your symptoms—or lack thereof—can cause you to fluctuate between feeling positive that the cycle has worked and being sure that it hasn't. These ups and downs are as common as the vast range of physical and emotional symptoms you may feel during this time.

If your obsession with symptoms is getting out of hand (also common!), try spending a little time each day jotting notes about what you are feeling in the Two-Week Wait Observation Log. The daily activity will help to pass the time, and writing your physical and emotional symptoms down on paper will give you a record of the previous day's experiences, so if you like, you can easily compare notes from earlier in the wait.

Mysterious twinges, cramps, sore breasts, food cravings, strange dreams, crankiness, and extreme exhaustion are just a few of the symptoms that might make your list, but no matter what your observances, just keep in mind that symptoms are not always representative of an actual result. Medications, elevated hormone levels, and procedural side effects along with the stress of an IVF cycle can mimic pregnancy and period symptoms, which—to make things even more confusing—are often the same. Furthermore, some women experience early pregnancy symptoms but many do not. The reality is that there is no way to tell if you are pregnant based solely on symptoms, but tracking them can be a positive outlet for dealing with the stress they can cause.

You also can also use The Two-Week Wait Observation Log to note any testing you may receive from your clinic, or any tests bought over-the-counter during the Two-Week Wait. There are conflicting schools of thought regarding the use of home pregnancy tests during the Two-Week Wait. Many experts and patients do not advocate their use, as they are not considered accurate predictors of pregnancy at such an early stage, and in an IVF cycle you run the risk of getting a false positive due to lingering HCG hormones from your trigger shot. Of course, the decision is yours; and if you are going to use home pregnancy tests, this log is where you would note the type, time, and result.

Finally, the Two-Week Wait Observation Log can be an extremely useful tool for the future. If your cycle is positive you will have a great record of early pregnancy. If your results are negative and you decide to cycle again, you will likely refer to this log many times during your next Two-Week Wait.

TWO-WEEK WAIT PROJECT PLANNER

Mood: Indulgent

Feel like pampering yourself? Whether your idea of pampering is a full spa day or reading a good book...go for it!

1. _____
2. _____
3. _____

Mood: Stressed

Deep breaths, bubble bath, a good stretch, yoga retreat, retail therapy... any option that calms you down is a good one!

1. _____
2. _____
3. _____

Mood: Productive

We all have things we want to do but always seem to put off, like a messy closet or a work project. Whatever it is, get it done!

1. _____
2. _____
3. _____

Mood: Philanthropic

Pass the time in a positive way by making an elderly neighbor some cookies or volunteering for a local cause.

1. _____
2. _____
3. _____

Mood: Tired

Rest is wonderful! There are lots of things you can do from the couch; write, surf the Web, play games and yes...just nap!

1. _____
2. _____
3. _____

Mood: Adventurous

Up for trying something new, like learning to knit? Straighten your hair? Make lobster bisque? Now is the time!

1. _____
2. _____
3. _____

Favorites

These are a few of my favorite things . . .

1. _____ 3. _____
2. _____ 4. _____

TWO-WEEK WAIT CALENDAR

Wait Day 1:

Wait Day 2:

Wait Day 3:

Wait Day 4:

Wait Day 5:

Wait Day 6:

Wait Day 7:

Wait Day 8:

Wait Day 9:

Wait Day 10:

Wait Day 11:

Wait Day 12:

Wait Day 13:

Wait Day 14:

TWO-WEEK WAIT OBSERVATION LOG

Date: _____ Cycle Day: _____

_____

_____

Date: _____ Cycle Day: _____

_____

_____

Date: _____ Cycle Day: _____

_____

_____

Date: _____ Cycle Day: _____

_____

_____

Date: _____ Cycle Day: _____

_____

_____

Date: _____ Cycle Day: _____

_____

_____

Date: _____ Cycle Day: _____

_____

_____

TWO-WEEK WAIT OBSERVATION LOG

Date: _____ Cycle Day: _____

_____

_____

Date: _____ Cycle Day: _____

_____

_____

Date: _____ Cycle Day: _____

_____

_____

Date: _____ Cycle Day: _____

_____

_____

Date: _____ Cycle Day: _____

_____

_____

Date: _____ Cycle Day: _____

_____

_____

Date: _____ Cycle Day: _____

_____

_____

Chapter 10
BALANCING ACT:
PREPPING FOR YOUR RESULTS

THE END OF what may feel like the longest two weeks of your life comes down to one day: Results Day. The best way to approach this major milestone is the same way you have approached your IVF treatment: by being informed and prepared. In the case of results, prepping involves two things: being careful to balance hope and reality (or being cautiously optimistic) and considering both possible cycle outcomes, positive and negative.

The sad reality is that not all IVF cycles work. Success rates vary based on many factors including age, clinic, treatment type, and diagnosis; but even under the best conditions there are no guarantees. Due to this fact, you can and should be hopeful, excited, and ready for wonderful news, but you must also be armed with facts and have a plan in place if the results are not good. Planning can't take away the pain of a negative result, but it can serve as a guide to help get you through what might otherwise be a very hard time.

This act of balancing hope and reality, or practicing cautious optimism, is not always easy during IVF. Stress and hormones, combined with everyday life, can cause your emotions to jump around constantly. You may have moments when you are sure the cycle worked, and low points where you feel sure that it did not. Prepping for your results can serve to alleviate some of those ups and downs and the stress that may be associated with the close of your cycle.

HOW TO USE THIS CHAPTER

This chapter provides worksheets designed to help you prepare for your results by prompting you to understand your testing procedure and outlining specific steps that you might take based on a negative or positive outcome. Understanding the facts about your results and testing phase is crucial, because any small hiccups during this critical period can make the stress mount and the wait feel even longer.

First, use the Pregnancy Test Prepping Worksheet to make sure you understand your pregnancy test procedure. Pregnancy tests for IVF, often referred to as beta tests, measure the amount of HCG in your blood, which is produced by the placenta shortly after the embryo attaches to the uterine lining. Start with the test basics: where, when, and what time. After you understand these, you can begin to get into specifics. Ask about the test procedure and whether there are any specific instructions. Is it a simple blood test or is there anything else involved? Some clinics use a two-day test system with one test on Day 10 or 12 and another two days later while some only perform one test. If you are on a two-day test system, do you get the results separately and immediately, or all at once after the second test?

Next, ask what you are being tested for and what qualifies as a positive result. Different clinics look for different HCG levels based on the actual day of the test, and unfortunately, pregnancy test results are not always black and white. You should ask your reproductive endocrinologist (RE) or nurse to review all possible outcomes, and you can review the IVF Basics section so you have a good understanding of outcomes that may fall into a gray area. You can also ask if they test for other post-cycle hormone levels, like progesterone.

After you understand what you are being tested for and what qualifies as a positive result, you can ask how and when you will be notified about your results. Even if it means waiting a bit longer to find out, set up a notification plan with your clinic that works for your schedule. If they cannot either give you an exact time or call you at a time that works for you, ask them to leave a message with the results at a specific number so that you can retrieve it on your own time.

As you set up your notification plan with your clinic, consider where you (and your partner) will be when you get the news and make a Results Day Plan. Nothing is worse than getting a call that delivers bad news during a work event or in the middle of a public place. If you cannot be at home together, make a plan to connect at a certain time or place where you both have access to private and comforting surroundings, should you need them.

OPTIMISM FIRST:
PREPPING FOR A POSITIVE

Preparing for positive results is probably something that you have been doing for some time. Picturing your baby and all the joy he or she will bring is a great way to stay positive throughout your cycle, and if you haven't already, you can begin to think about a special way to celebrate with your partner and tell your family and friends the good news. Just make sure not to break the bank or go overboard with details until you have an official result.

You probably already know the color of the baby's room and your favorite brand of maternity jeans, but when prepping for a positive you must consider some practical IVF questions as well. Use the Continued Treatment and Care box on the Positive Results Prepping Worksheet to answer the following questions: How does your clinic handle post-positive monitoring and testing? Will they perform regular blood work and ultrasounds or immediately release you to your OB/GYN? What physical milestones and levels do they use to confirm a healthy pregnancy? What medications or supplements will you continue on or start to take, and for how long? Most clinics recommend continued progesterone support, so you will need to make sure you can refill your prescription in a timely manner based on your results. No matter what you do, plan to celebrate, relax, and enjoy the moment. You certainly will have earned it!

ERRING ON THE SIDE OF CAUTION:
PREPPING FOR A NEGATIVE

Preparing for negative results is a bit more complicated than positive prepping, but it is still extremely important. If you don't have a plan, receiving a negative result can feel like stepping off a cliff with no warning. Preparing cannot take away the pain of the fall, but it can help to support you on your climb back up. Right now, it may seem unnecessary to actually write these things down, but if you get a negative result, having a concrete guide right in front of you that you can follow without thinking is extremely helpful and comforting.

Use the Negative Results Prepping Worksheet to make a short list of immediate steps to take if you get a negative result. These steps can be as simple or as intricate as you feel comfortable with and can include writing a venting entry in your journal or taking a few days off to mourn and recover your physical and emotional strength. A change of scenery can help you process the news, and help you to reach a place where you are ready to face the realities of your results. If time off is not an option, try pre-booking a massage, yoga class or therapy session. Even if you don't go, the option will be there if it feels right. If you have a therapist, mentor, or cycle buddy, plan a time and place to connect with them; or, simply have your iPod ready with soothing music or meditations.

Next, think longer term about some activities that can help get you through the weeks and months following your cycle. You may find comfort in getting right back on the horse and researching treatments, clinics, and next steps, or you might prefer to take a mental and physical break. If you want to take your mind off treatment, try planning a large project that will carry you through a long period of time. Starting a garden or home renovation, getting a pet, researching new career paths, planning a vacation, or organizing a large event are all good ideas.

Finally, think about your overall fertility plan, all the while knowing that you can always change your mind, any time you want. Discuss your options with your partner and think about how you will feel and react to bad news. If the outcome of this cycle is negative, will you cycle again right away or take some time off? Will you decide to try alternative treatments or look into donor or adoption paths? What are your options? Your preferences?

There are many wonderful resources for support before, during, and after your cycle. If you haven't already, spend some of that pent up energy from your Two-Week Wait researching your options for support. The list of non-profit and fertility organizations on pages 159–161 can point you in the right direction, and Chapter 13 provides more space to organize your personal support network and support resources.

PREGNANCY TEST PREPPING WORKSHEET

Pregnancy Test Details

Test Day: _____   Test Time: _____   Location: _____

Procedure/ Instructions: _____

_____

_____

_____

Hormones Tested: _____

_____

_____

_____

Desired Levels: _____

_____

_____

_____

Notification Details/Call Plan: _____

_____

_____

_____

Results Day Plan: _____

_____

_____

_____

POSITIVE RESULTS PREPPING WORKSHEET

Celebration and Announcement Plans:

_____

_____

_____

_____

Continued Treatment and Care:

Post-Positive Monitoring and Test Information: _____

_____

_____

_____

Healthy Pregnancy Milestones: _____

_____

_____

_____

Post-Positive Medication Information: _____

_____

_____

_____

Release Date to OB/GYN: _____

_____

_____

_____

NEGATIVE RESULTS PREPPING WORKSHEET

Immediate Coping Steps: _____

_____

_____

_____

_____

_____

Longer Term Coping Steps: _____

_____

_____

_____

_____

_____

Overall Fertility Plan/Options for Moving Forward: _____

_____

_____

_____

_____

_____

Support Resources: _____

_____

_____

_____

_____

Chapter 11

DEALING WITH YOUR RESULTS

THIS CHAPTER COVERS both negative and positive results and is designed to be used after you receive your results. My wish is that no one ever needs the negative results pages. However, negative results are a reality for many patients, and my hope is that this section provides information, comfort, and support for those who must face that reality.

Feel free to read about both outcomes in advance, but if it feels more comfortable, you can also wait and read only the result that applies to you. If you receive a negative result, my advice is that you do not reread the positive results pages; if need be, ask your partner or a friend to remove them.

A NEGATIVE RESULT

If you are facing a negative result, know that my heart is breaking for you. There are no words, no consolation, and nothing fair about a failed cycle, but please know that for most people, the pain of a negative result does ease with time, and you will not always feel like this.

Right now you may be reeling from weeks or months of hormones, medications, tests, dashed hope, despair, anger, and sadness. However you respond to this pain is absolutely fine. It is extremely normal to need and want help, so please consider the options available. Turn to your partner, family members, friends, a private therapist, a support group, or to the organizations listed on pages 159–161. Do whatever you need to in order to take care of yourself.

If this was your first cycle, you may find comfort in the fact that oftentimes the first IVF cycle is thought of as a trial run. It is very difficult to know how you will respond to the procedures and medications, so a failed cycle can be a learning experience and a way for your medical team to further diagnose your infertility. If that isn't the case and they didn't find a reason for your negative outcome, take solace in the fact that even Mother Nature only has about a 25 percent success rate for women *without* fertility problems.

If you used the Negative Results Prepping Worksheet, go back and review it as soon as possible. Even if it feels impossible, try starting with one thing on the list. If the plans you made don't feel right or comfortable now, try to come up with some new options that fit your current state of mind. If you are having a hard time moving forward, just keep in mind that it is very common to feel exhausted and numb after a negative result. It's perfectly acceptable to do nothing for a few days as well. Just make sure that you seek professional help if you find yourself in a persistent funk, or if you are experiencing signs of depression.

Whenever you feel ready you should schedule a follow-up call or appointment with your reproductive endocrinologist (RE). The follow-up call should cover a review of your treatment plan and protocol, the results of each phase of the cycle, and your response to the medications and procedures. If you like, you can review your notes to see if you have general or specific questions relating to any test, procedure, or response. You should discuss the possible reasons that the cycle failed, but keep in mind that there is often no clear answer as to why cycles fail.

Also plan to discuss options for moving forward based on your diagnosis and the information learned in this cycle. If this was not your first cycle, or if you plan on cycling again, you should also discuss your progress or any recommended changes to your treatment and protocol. You can also use the Multiple Cycles section to help you as you move forward with treatment.

Most importantly, take the next few days and weeks slowly, and really try to focus on healing yourself.

Date and Time of Follow-Up Appointment or Call: _____

_____

Protocol and Review of Cycle Phases: _____

_____

_____

_____

Medications, Response and Procedure Review: _____

_____

_____

_____

Possible Reasons for Failure: _____

_____

_____

_____

_____

Options for Moving Forward: _____

_____

_____

_____

_____

A POSITIVE RESULT

Congratulations are (finally!) in order, and you have definitely earned them! You have worked hard and persevered through a very difficult time and can finally begin the journey of your pregnancy. The emotions you may have during an IVF pregnancy will be much like those of a normal pregnancy, and for many women who conceive through IVF the sense of relief and accomplishment serves to enhance the experience.

On the flip side, every new pregnancy comes with some level of worry and trepidation, and for those who have suffered from infertility or previous loss, these feelings can be magnified. There are great resources available for women who become pregnant through IVF or other infertility treatments. If you feel as though you would benefit from some extra support, check out the organizations on pages 159–161, as they often have resources related to pregnancy after infertility. If you can't find a resource, ask your fertility clinic or OB/GYN for suggestions.

If you haven't already, you can now figure out your potential due date and the timing of your trimesters based on the completed cycle. One way to estimate your due date is to add 38 weeks to the day of your egg retrieval. This is based on the traditional method of setting a due date at 40 weeks from the first day of your last period. Of course this is not scientific, and you should rely on your OB/GYN for a specific due date, but it is very fun!

Logistically you will still have a few hurdles to get through before you are released from your clinic's care. These usually include a series of tests measuring your HCG levels, and an ultrasound somewhere between 5 and 8 weeks. Review your Positive Results Prepping Worksheet and use the Positive Results Follow-Up Worksheet to record these results.

If everything goes well, you will likely be released from your IVF clinic to a general OB/GYN sometime during your first trimester. This switch can be a bit unsettling as you reenter life as a mainstream patient, but just remember: the end of one road is the beginning of another, and you should continue to empower and advocate for yourself throughout pregnancy and motherhood the same way you have throughout the IVF process.

As an IVF pregnancy you are one of the lucky few that know they are pregnant right from the get-go. So, if you wish, the Two-Week Wait Observation Log and other sections of this book can now serve as a memento of early pregnancy and your unique road to achieving it. Enjoy!

POSITIVE RESULTS FOLLOW-UP WORKSHEET

Estimating Your Due Date

Egg Retrieval Date: _____ + 38 Weeks = Estimated Due Date: _____

Follow-Up Testing

Date	HCG Level	Progesterone	Ultrasound Results	Notes

Notes: _____

_____

_____

_____

_____

SECTION VI
SUPPORT
FOR MIND
AND BODY

Chapter 12

SELF-AWARENESS: SURVIVING THE IVF ROLLERCOASTER

FOR GOOD REASON, infertility and IVF cycles are often compared to roller-coaster rides, and whether or not you are a coaster fan, your cycle may have some (or many) ups and downs. During your cycle you may feel hope, excitement, determination, disappointment, loss, joy, exhaustion, stress, and much more, sometimes all at the same time!

Don't worry, this is par for the course during a cycle, and believe me: this crazy roller-coaster ride is enough to send even the strongest of us spinning. The good news is that with a little effort you can learn to look for the curves and hills ahead, so you will know when to hold on a bit tighter and call in some extra support, and when it is safe to relax and throw your hands up.

Anticipating ups and downs (and thus surviving the IVF roller coaster) starts with self-awareness. Being self-aware means noticing and acknowledging your emotions and resulting moods—including what causes them and how you react to them. Doing this helps you keep things in perspective so you can get and stay positive and cope during difficult times.

For instance, when you notice that you are in a particularly bad mood, practicing self-awareness can help you figure out why you are upset. If you understand why you are upset, you have a better shot at finding a solution to your problem and avoiding it next time. When you can't avoid stressful situations, the simple act of being aware of them can help reduce their negative impact. Being blindsided by a stressful situation can make it harder to recover from but if you know you are about to be thrown for a loop you can hold on tighter and take that loop in stride. Similarly, by noticing your positive emotions you will be able to recognize, re-create, and call on positive influences and events when you need a little (or big!) boost.

Remember, even if you are not a roller-coaster fan, practicing self-awareness will give you a good chance of getting off this crazy ride without losing your lunch!

JOURNALING YOUR WAY TO SELF-AWARENESS

Journaling is a great way to develop self-awareness. Not only does it provide a concrete record of past events but it is a safe, easy, inexpensive way to reduce stress and release pent up emotions. It helps you to reach a deeper level of personal understanding by holding your thoughts and feelings still so that you can consider them objectively.

If you already journal, then keep at it; the benefits are limitless, especially as you go through IVF. If you have never tried it, just remember that the key to successful journaling is finding a method that works for you. Journaling does not have to be the traditional "Dear Diary" format that many people expect. It can include daily entries, random thoughts, one-word observations, drawings, doodles, magazine clippings, or personal photos, lists, and more. For example, my journal is not a narrative where I write or speak to a third party about myself, my experiences, and my feelings. I instead simply write my thoughts and feelings down in an unstructured, bullet-point style list that includes events, feelings, rants, raves, and just about anything else. Some of my bullet points are one word, others are pages long.

Another idea is to write directly to the person or issue you are thinking about. You can even write directly to your emotions, as a way to flush out what you are feeling. Write to your fear and frustration; ask questions, offer solutions, excuses, and alternatives. Write to yourself or your friends, your family or your providers. You may be surprised at what you learn. You will also find yourself able to:

· Clarify thoughts, feelings, behaviors, desires, and needs

· Strengthen your sense of self

- Reveal and track patterns and cycles, helping you better cope with mood swings and stress

- Build self-confidence and self-knowledge

- Identify what is important so you can stay focused on the positive

- Gain new perspective and connect to the bigger picture

- Make decision making easier

- Provide insight into what makes you happy, sad, angry, or frustrated

- Shed light on and therefore improve your relationship with others

The end of this book includes blank journal pages to get you started, so give it a try. I bet you will be glad you did!

HOW TO USE THIS CHAPTER

The IVF Emotion Log is designed to help you practice self-awareness by tracking your emotions throughout your cycle. Use this as frequently as you like; as you mark your moods, jot down a note as to their cause. When things are not great, you will have a better understanding of why and can try to rectify things if you so desire. You will also be more aware of and better able to recognize positives, which are sometimes easy to forget or ignore. You can also use the IVF Emotion Log to see whether your emotions (good and bad) may have some correlation to procedures, medications, or complementary therapies. This is not only interesting to track but can provide great insight toward helping you better manage your ups and downs in the future.

As you work on self-awareness, build your support network and use complementary therapies, it is inevitable that you will come across a lot of different types of advice along the way. Some of this advice might be very useful, some not so much so. Always remember there is no such thing as universal advice—different things work for different people. The IVF Tips and Advice page provides a place where you can note any advice you have received along the way that you would like to try or remember.

Cycle Day Date/Time	Mood					Notes
	Very Low	Low	Level	Good	Very Good	

IVF TIPS AND ADVICE

Source: _____

Advice or Tip: _____

_____

_____

_____

Source: _____

Advice or Tip: _____

_____

_____

_____

Source: _____

Advice or Tip: _____

_____

_____

_____

Source: _____

Advice or Tip: _____

_____

_____

_____

Chapter 13

Don't Go It Alone: Complementary Therapies and a Support Network

THE IVF PROCESS is not always easy, and having access to your own personal support network is a great way to stay positive, informed, and connected during your treatment. It is also a great comfort to know you have go-to resources when you are faced with difficulties, whether it's a small bump in the road or a larger emotional or physical crisis.

There are loads of resources available for women going through infertility and IVF, so spend a little time researching and determining which options you are most comfortable with. Some popular options include complementary or alternative therapies; peer support and discussion groups; private, group or couples therapy; as well as books, websites, social media communities, blogs, and message boards. Many patients also turn to family and friends, or have a cycle buddy or mentor—someone who is currently going through or has been through IVF treatment and understands the journey you are on.

As you consider your options, keep in mind that your support network should provide you with resources that not only educate and inform but also help you feel connected and comforted while you go through treatment. Strong resources help offer emotional relief by providing opportunities for you to soothe yourself in whatever way you are most comfortable with. They also help you:

- Explore and vent your feelings—including unsettling ones

- Learn and gather information

- Make decisions—both large and small

- Develop coping skills

- Mourn loss and celebrate success

- Relax physically and emotionally

Complementary therapies are a great form of support for IVF patients and can greatly enhance your experience. They can help you to reduce stress and feel more relaxed and can improve your physical and emotional health as well. They also provide positive ways to pass the time during a cycle, especially during waiting periods.

Some popular options include mind and body programs, yoga, meditation and visualization, acupuncture and massage. If you are employing or interested in exploring these or other options, start by asking your clinic and other contacts for information and referrals, or use the organizations and contacts in your support network to search for practitioners in your area. You can also turn to the National Center for Complementary and Alternative Medicine. This is a United States government resource and a good place to research your options. Their information can be found at www.nccam.nih.gov.

No matter what type of practice you are considering, most therapies have different styles, pricing, and practitioners available. To get the most out of any treatment, you should feel comfortable with all aspects of the program, including price, location, schedule, and instructor or technician.

It is important to note that complementary therapies can provide great benefits for some, but if a certain practice is not your cup of tea, then you should not feel compelled to use it. If you are doing something that you don't enjoy, the stress of stress relief can ironically do more harm than good. You should only do what you feel comfortable with, and if that does not include complementary therapies, then you should not feel obligated to pursue them.

HOW TO USE THIS CHAPTER

This chapter includes a Resources Worksheet which prompts you to put together your own personal support network. If at all possible, try to work on this section as soon as you can, as there are many uses for it before, during, and after your cycle. Resources, including complementary therapies, should be about quality, not quantity; however, as you move through your cycle, your needs may change. If possible, try to give yourself a few different options for support; but if you end up with only a few, that is fine as well.

Start the process of considering your options for support by jotting down notes about what you already consider to be important resources. These can include any valuable sources of information on infertility and IVF, as well as any places where you have found support or information thus far. Next ask your clinic contacts and other providers if they recommend any support options.

A great way to start building your support network is to review and explore the Non-Profit and Fertility Organizations on pages 159–161. As you research, fill in the Support Network Worksheets with organizations that appeal to you and have a presence in your area, or that you can easily access via the Web. Check to see if they offer support groups, educational programs, events, or information on topics that concern or interest you, and which relate to your specific treatment and diagnosis.

Next, consider the people who support you. Make a list of any close friends or family members who are a go-to for support when you need it and if you have a cycle buddy or a mentor whom you are sharing your journey with include their info as well.

If you are already working with, or interested in exploring private mental health practitioners, add their information to the Support Network Worksheets. Most clinics have on-staff counselors or therapists or provide referrals to professionals trained in infertility counseling. Even if you think you won't need this type of resource it doesn't hurt to have it *just in case*.

Next make a list of your favorite online resources, including websites, twitter feeds, blogs, social media communities, and the like. Add to that any books that you like, noting pages that you may want to find in a hurry and voilà—your personal support network is complete!

If part of your support system includes complementary therapies, use the Complementary Therapy Options Worksheet to explore, document, and organize your options. Make sure you understand the treatment, program, cost, and basic details. Whether you practice yoga every day or try acupuncture once, you can evaluate and track your response, both emotional and physical, with the Complementary Therapy Log.

Infertility and IVF can be isolating and it is not uncommon to feel alone as you go through treatment. So while it may seem unnecessary to actually write down this type of information, give it a try—just seeing your support network in writing not only provides comfort and boosts your confidence but also makes it more likely that you will ask for (and therefore receive) support when you need it.

RESOURCES WORKSHEET

Favorite Resources:

_____

_____

_____

_____

_____

_____

_____

_____

_____

_____

Clinic and Provider Recommendations:

_____

_____

_____

_____

_____

_____

_____

_____

_____

SUPPORT NETWORK WORKSHEET

Favorite Organizations:

Organization: _____

Web Address: _____ Phone / Hotline: _____

Programs / Event Info: _____

_____

_____

Organization: _____

Web Address: _____ Phone / Hotline: _____

Programs / Event Info: _____

_____

_____

Local Support Group Information:

Held By: _____ Meeting Time: _____

Location: _____

Information /Description: _____

My People (Cycle Buddies, Mentors, Therapist, Family Friends):

Name: _____ Phone: _____ Email: _____

Name: _____ Phone: _____ Email: _____

Name: _____ Phone: _____ Email: _____

Name: _____ Phone: _____ Email: _____

Name: _____ Phone: _____ Email: _____

Name: _____ Phone: _____ Email: _____

SUPPORT NETWORK WORKSHEET

Favorite Web Resources:

Site: _____

    Username: _____ Password: _____

Site: _____

    Username: _____ Password: _____

Site: _____

    Username: _____ Password: _____

Site: _____

    Username: _____ Password: _____

Site: _____

    Username: _____ Password: _____

Favorite Books:

Book: _____

    Author: _____ Notable Pages: _____

Book: _____

    Author: _____ Notable Pages: _____

Book: _____

    Author: _____ Notable Pages: _____

Book: _____

    Author: _____ Notable Pages: _____

Book: _____

    Author: _____ Notable Pages: _____

COMPLEMENTARY THERAPY OPTIONS WORKSHEET

Company: _____ Contact: _____ Phone: _____

Email: _____ Website: _____

Address: _____ City: _____ State: _____ Zip: _____

Practice Type & Overview: _____

_____

Hours / Schedule / Class Times: _____

_____

Company Policy Notes: _____

Treatment Costs: _____

Company: _____ Contact: _____ Phone: _____

Email: _____ Website: _____

Address: _____ City: _____ State: _____ Zip: _____

Practice Type & Overview: _____

_____

Hours / Schedule / Class Times: _____

_____

Company Policy Notes: _____

Treatment Costs: _____

Company: _____ Contact: _____ Phone: _____

Email: _____ Website: _____

Address: _____ City: _____ State: _____ Zip: _____

Practice Type & Overview: _____

_____

Hours / Schedule / Class Times: _____

_____

Company Policy Notes: _____

Treatment Costs: _____

COMPLEMENTARY THERAPY LOG

Date & Time:	Therapy Details:	Observances:

Date & Time:	Therapy Details:	Observances:

Date & Time:	Therapy Details:	Observances:

Date & Time:	Therapy Details:	Observances:

Date & Time:	Therapy Details:	Observances:

Date & Time:	Therapy Details:	Observances:

SECTION VII
MULTIPLE CYCLES

Chapter 14

Off to the Races, Again: Multiple Cycles and FET's

IF YOU ARE about to embark on your second cycle or have undergone multiple rounds of IVF, you already know that multiple cycles come with their own set of challenges and concerns. Each new round of IVF can bring an unsettling mix of emotions as you attempt to move past your previous loss and focus on the present. As you move through treatment it is likely that you will want to compare procedures, responses, and other notable events from one cycle to the next and you may be looking for progress in specific areas by trying new medications, procedures, or therapies each time. Whether you are on your second, third or fourth cycle, tracking and organizing information can provide a wealth of data and great peace of mind.

For some patients their second or subsequent cycles are Frozen Embryo Transfers (FET). This means you have frozen embryos from a previous cycle that will be thawed and then transferred into your uterus. An FET is sort of like a half-cycle, and while no less emotional, many patients find that FETs are physically and logistically easier than regular cycles. While you will likely take medications before, during, and after the cycle, there are usually fewer medications and appointments because you skip the stimulation, egg retrieval, and embryo growth phases.

It is important to note that not all frozen embryos "survive the thaw." In many cases multiple embryos are defrosted, but not all will be suitable for transfer. If you have a low number of frozen embryos, you may be in a position where you won't know until the last minute whether you will be able to have your transfer. Because of this, most clinics will give you a set time for transfer, but will also call you the morning of the transfer (your embryos will have defrosted overnight) to confirm that your procedure is a go. The night before your scheduled procedure can be a long one, and the resulting disappointment can be difficult to bear if none of your thawed embryos are suitable for transfer. Talk to your reproductive endocrinologist (RE) and embryologist about your specific situation, including how many embryos you have total, and how many they plan to defrost to get a viable embryo. Also, make sure you understand the call plan: know when you are due to the clinic and when you will get the call. If you travel for treatment, this can be tricky, and you may have to leave before you know the results of the thaw, or move quickly once you know the transfer is a go.

LET'S GET THIS PARTY STARTED: A SPECIAL RITUAL FOR MULTI-CYCLERS

When you are facing a second (or third or fourth!) treatment cycle, it can be easy to focus on the negative and to become overwhelmed by the sheer fact that you have to do it all over again. My advice is to honor the journey you are on by having a little commemoration ceremony at the start of your cycle. I did and it made me feel a whole lot better.

After recovering from the pain and loss of a failed cycle, and as my new cycle approached, I remained hopeful, happy, and really excited to try again. But as excited as I was, when it came time to take that first shot or pill, the waterworks would start. And when I say waterworks, I mean the flood gates would open. I was hit hard by the realization that not only was I still not pregnant but also that I had to do it all again, and that I had to go to such great lengths to achieve something most of my peers achieved naturally, or with only one try at IVF.

Because I had experienced it all before, some of the fear of the unknown had dissipated, but mostly I felt overwhelmed and exhausted. The process of treatment—the shots, the tests, the appointments, the procedures, the hope, the hormones, and of course, the potential disappointment—all loomed large. In my low moments it looked like a mountain that I just couldn't climb again. I knew that an emotional low point was not where I wanted to be when I started a cycle. I knew that something had to change. I wanted and needed to hold on to the positive energy, hope, and excitement that we often feel when starting treatment, so it could carry me through another cycle.

That is when my husband and I started our "Cycle Commemoration Ceremony." Ours was a slightly silly, simple ritual, usually performed in the vicinity of the bedroom or bathroom. We would sit and look at the medications laid out before us again and have a bit of a pep talk and congratulations speech all in one. It went a little something like this: We acknowledged that we were at the beginning again, and that we were ready to fight this battle together. Next, we admitted that it wasn't going to be easy and allowed ourselves to be proud of the fact that we had the strength to do it again. We recognized the sadness and the hope that came with starting a new cycle and with the toast-like clink of syringes we were on our way. Eventually the waterworks were replaced with a few glistening tears, and finally, with a strength and a resolve that I never knew I possessed.

So whatever you consider to be the start of your next cycle, and however you chose to do it, take some time to mark the moment, mourn the loss that comes with a failed cycle, and give your next cycle and yourself due credit. A pre-cycle pep talk might do the job for you, or it might be a mini-vacation, a night out to dinner, or another personal ritual that bolsters your spirit and your confidence. Whatever it is, go ahead—you have earned it!

HOW TO USE THIS CHAPTER

Depending on where you are in your treatment you can use this chapter in conjunction with the rest of the book or on its own. If you are in a cycle (not your first) you can use the other sections of the book to record your current cycle and fill the charts in this chapter with data from your previous cycle(s) by requesting a copy of your medical records from your clinic. Using the charts in this chapter together can help you to draw a correlation between your medications, stimulation results, and procedural responses.

The chapter begins with a Cycle to Cycle Comparison Chart that allows you to compare the basics of up to four cycles, side by side. This is a good way to see a broad overview of your journey, while the charts that follow will allow you to compare more specific details.

The Stimulation Medication Comparison Chart allows you to see how many days you "stimmed" for during each cycle and what type and dose of medication you took each day. To use the chart, mark the cycle number at the top of each column and fill in the dose and type of stimulation medication you took on each day of stimulation. If you like you can also use this chart to note the day and details (time, medication type, and dose) of your trigger shot by simply changing the box after your last stimulation day to Trigger Shot Day.

The Stimulation Results Comparison Chart tracks the basics of your stimulation phase. Each box should be used for one cycle. You can note the cycle day that your monitoring appointments fell on, and the basic results for each test, such as the number of follicles you had that day, your estrogen level and what your uterine lining looked like. Use the Comparison Notes section for any other information or observances you want to record and compare.

The Retrieval and Transfer Comparison Chart covers egg retrieval, semen samples, embryo growth, and transfer information.

The Post-Cycle Review Worksheets provide space for you to review and reflect, both on the previous cycle and the one to come. Use this space and the Multiple Cycle Notes Page that follows to document information from your providers, updates on your diagnosis, newly suggested testing, reasons your RE may have given you for your results, and what their plans are for moving forward. Finally, document any plans you may have for the next cycle, such as provider, medication, or treatment plan changes, or any new complementary therapy techniques you may be employing.

Cycling more than once is not easy, and it can be extremely difficult to muster up the strength and determination to cycle again. As you move through treatment, take heart and remember there are benefits that come with having cycled before. Simply being aware of the process of an IVF cycle can remove some of the unknowns and make subsequent cycles easier to navigate. Previous cycles can also provide a greater understanding of your diagnosis and treatment, which you can use to more confidently face the challenges that lie ahead.

CYCLE TO CYCLE COMPARISON CHART

	Cycle #:	Cycle #:	Cycle #:	Cycle #:
Date				
Clinic				
Reproductive Endocrinologist (RE)				
Protocol				
Medications				
Total Follicles				
Eggs Retrieved				
Eggs Fertilized				
Embryo(s) Transferred				
Embryo(s) Frozen				
Cycle Result				

STIMULATION MEDICATION COMPARISON CHART

	Cycle #:	Cycle #:	Cycle #:	Cycle #:
Stimulation Day #1				
Stimulation Day #2				
Stimulation Day #3				
Stimulation Day #4				
Stimulation Day #5				
Stimulation Day #6				
Stimulation Day #7				
Stimulation Day #8				
Stimulation Day #9				
Stimulation Day #10				
Stimulation Day #11				
Stimulation Day #12				

STIMULATION RESULTS COMPARISON CHART

Cycle #	Cycle Day	Follicles	Lining	Estradiol	Other
1st Monitoring					
2nd Monitoring					
3rd Monitoring					
4th Monitoring					
5th Monitoring					

Comparison Notes

Cycle #	Cycle Day	Follicles	Lining	Estradiol	Other
1st Monitoring					
2nd Monitoring					
3rd Monitoring					
4th Monitoring					
5th Monitoring					

Comparison Notes

Cycle #	Cycle Day	Follicles	Lining	Estradiol	Other
1st Monitoring					
2nd Monitoring					
3rd Monitoring					
4th Monitoring					
5th Monitoring					

Comparison Notes

Cycle #	Cycle Day	Follicles	Lining	Estradiol	Other
1st Monitoring					
2nd Monitoring					
3rd Monitoring					
4th Monitoring					
5th Monitoring					

Comparison Notes

	Cycle #:	Cycle #:	Cycle #:	Cycle #:
Eggs Retrieved/Mature				
Sperm Volume				
Sperm Motility				
Sperm Morphology				
Sperm Concentration				
Egg Fertilized				
Embryos on Day 2				
Embryos on Day 3				
Embryos on Day 4				
Embryos Transferred				
Embryos Frozen				

POST-CYCLE REVIEW WORKSHEET

Cycle #: ___ Cycle Date: _____ Protocol: _____

RE Response: _____

_____

_____

Protocol Recommendations for Next Cycle: _____

_____

_____

Post-Cycle Testing Recommendations: _____

_____

_____

Results: _____

_____

_____

_____

Feelings about This Cycle: _____

_____

_____

Personal Plans for Next Cycle: _____

_____

_____

_____

POST-CYCLE REVIEW WORKSHEET

Cycle #: ___ Cycle Date: _____ Protocol: _____

RE Response: _____

_____

_____

Protocol Recommendations for Next Cycle: _____

_____

_____

Post-Cycle Testing Recommendations: _____

_____

_____

Results: _____

_____

_____

_____

Feelings about This Cycle: _____

_____

_____

Personal Plans for Next Cycle: _____

_____

_____

_____

POST-CYCLE REVIEW WORKSHEET

Cycle #: ___ Cycle Date: _____ Protocol: _____

RE Response: _____

_____

_____

Protocol Recommendations for Next Cycle: _____

_____

_____

Post-Cycle Testing Recommendations: _____

_____

_____

Results: _____

_____

_____

_____

Feelings about This Cycle: _____

_____

_____

Personal Plans for Next Cycle: _____

_____

_____

_____

POST-CYCLE REVIEW WORKSHEET

Cycle #: ___ Cycle Date: _____ Protocol: _____

RE Response: _____

_____

_____

Protocol Recommendations for Next Cycle: _____

_____

_____

Post-Cycle Testing Recommendations: _____

_____

_____

Results: _____

_____

_____

_____

Feelings about This Cycle: _____

_____

_____

Personal Plans for Next Cycle: _____

_____

_____

_____

MULTIPLE CYCLE NOTES

CLOSING

A Note from the Author

Dear Readers,

Thank you for letting me accompany you during your cycle. IVF can be easy and quick for some, but for others it can be extremely difficult. For me it wasn't easy; in fact, it felt downright impossible at times. Writing this book, becoming a part of *your* process, saved me. For that I will be forever grateful.

I came up with the idea for *The IVF Journal* in January of 2009 during the Two-Week Wait of my second IVF cycle, but I really began writing it in September of 2005. After 45 two-week waits, one major surgery, 5 IUI cycles, and one IVF cycle resulting in a chemical pregnancy, my diagnosis was still the same: The dreaded "Unexplained Infertility."

During the Two-Week Wait of my next cycle, I was waiting, impatiently of course, and wishing I had a record of what my previous two-week waits had felt like. Since I had gotten pregnant during my first IVF cycle and did have early symptoms, I was going crazy trying to remember what day they occurred or how severe they were. So I started keeping a record of my symptoms.

When the cycle failed, I was, of course, distraught. I had responded much better to the medications this time compared to my previous cycles; I even made 20, yes *20* eggs! But I couldn't remember: how many eggs did I have during the last cycle when I actually became pregnant? What size were they? What grade did my embryos get?

It was then I decided: no more wondering. I knew I would cycle again and this time I was going to take control of the one thing I could—knowledge about myself, my body, my cycles, and my feelings. A small victory, but I'll take it. So *The IVF Journal* was born. Excuse the pun, but at least something was! First a simple calendar, then some charts, folders, and soon I had my very own IVF trapper keeper. Yeah, I like this. I thought that other IVFers might like this, too. Throughout the rest of my IVF treatment I worked on (and with) what has become *The IVF Journal*. Finally, after two more cycles and an FET, I found success and began the journey of motherhood and healing that has culminated in my sharing this book with you. I hope using *The IVF Journal* will help you as much as writing it for you helped me.

I commend your strength; I sympathize deeply with your heartaches and understand completely if you someday decide to throw this book in the trash. You might then dig it out again, only to chuck it once more! But in the end, I hope that it will become a memento of your unique story of bravery and strength on the way to motherhood.

With love and thanks,

Stephanie Fry

Acknowledgements

IT TOOK ME nearly ten years to live and write this book. Throughout that time my husband stood with me through round after round of treatment. He was by my side through loss, failure, resilience, resolution, hope, and despair. He not only stood with me, he often, quite literally, held me up. Russell, there are not words to thank you. You have been my sounding board, proofreader, financier, editor, guinea pig, nurse, therapist, logo designer, Web master, coach, teacher, cheerleader, and advocate. You have been, are, and always will be *everything*.

I'm also so grateful for the amazing group of women who were the first IVF patients to read, test, and provide feedback for what is now *The IVF Journal*. Erin, Crystal, Marianne, Leisha, Kathryn, Mary, Paivi and Sonia: Thank you for sharing your time, your stories and your insights. I am honored that you did so.

Dave: My fellow outlaw, my Brother-In-Law extraordinaire. Thank you for working for pennies and pats on the back and for quietly listening to years worth of rants and status updates without judgment or question—I needed it more than you may know. You brought color and style to my work, and without you *The IVF Journal* would never be what it is today.

Caroline and Evan, thank you both for taking the time to read the early versions of the book—you were the best pre-editors a girl could ask for! And, many thanks to Christopher and Heidi Harting; your expertise and generosity were a huge help in the beginning of this project.

And to my village, who over the past ten years made all this possible—Mom, Dad, Mel, Dear, Pop, Christie, Courtney, Laura, Becky, my girls, and the many amazing healthcare professionals who not only helped me overcome infertility but also helped to heal my mind—thank you. Thank you. Thank you!

Finally, to everyone at Hatherleigh Press especially Andrew Flach, Ryan Kennedy, and Anna Krusinski, a million thank-you's for seeing the value of this project and for taking my work to the next level. The work that you do is amazing and I am thrilled to be a part of it.

Non-Profit and Fertility Organizations

THERE ARE NUMEROUS organizations dedicated to fertility and everything it encompasses. Depending on your specific situation and needs, these groups can be wonderful resources that help you find information and referrals, connect with others in a similar situation, get educated about diagnoses and treatment, and cope with the stresses infertility and resulting treatments can bring.

Most organizations have a Web presence and many have local, in-person options for connecting as well. Options can include educational events, support groups, fertility trade shows, walks and more. There are hundreds of organizations in the United States and other countries that cover a wide range of infertility topics including IVF. Below are a few of my personal favorites.

RESOLVE, THE NATIONAL INFERTILITY ORGANIZATION (WWW.RESOLVE.ORG) AND RESOLVE NEW ENGLAND (WWW.RESOLVENEWENGLAND.ORG)

The RESOLVE organizations are the longest running non-profit organizations dedicated to fertility in the United States. Established in 1974, both organizations work tirelessly to improve the lives of people living with infertility by providing education, advocacy, and support. They both offer local in-person support groups, insurance hotlines, educational and other events, regular conference calls, and services that provide information on every aspect of infertility. Their websites and social media sites are great for finding links to local in-person support, medical information, emotional support, advocacy information, advocacy efforts, and much more.

RESOLVE. The National Infertility Association has a network that includes the Great Lakes Region, Mid-Atlantic Region, Midwest Region, Mountain Region, Northeast Region, North Pacific Region, South Central Region, Southeast Region, and Southwest Region.

RESOLVE New England serves the infertility community in the greater New England region, including Connecticut, Maine, Massachusetts, New Hampshire, Rhode Island, and Vermont.

THE AMERICAN FERTILITY ASSOCIATION
(WWW.THEAFA.ORG)

The American Fertility Association (The AFA) is another great U.S.-based non-profit organization that focuses on supporting people going through infertility. Headquartered in New York, they offer local and national programs that include educational outreach events, an online library, a resource directory, telephone and in-person coaching, and a toll-free support line. Their website and social media sites are also great places to find medical information, emotional support, advocacy information, advocacy efforts, and much more.

THE AMERICAN SOCIETY FOR REPRODUCTIVE MEDICINE
(WWW.ASRM.ORG)

The American Society for Reproductive Medicine (ASRM) describes itself as a multidisciplinary organization dedicated to the advancement of the art, science, and practice of reproductive medicine. They provide education and research and advocate on behalf of patients, physicians, and healthcare providers. Among other things, their services include educational events for medical professionals who are working in the field of reproductive medicine. For IVF patients and anyone dealing with infertility, their website www.reproductivefacts.org is a wonderful resource for medical information and includes downloadable Patient Fact Sheets and Booklets and one of the best infertility "Topics Index(es)" on the Web.

THE SOCIETY FOR ASSISTED REPRODUCTIVE TECHNOLOGY
(WWW.SART.ORG)

The Society for Assisted Reproductive Technology (SART) is an organization of professionals dedicated to the practice of Assisted Reproductive Technologies in the United States. They provide a wealth of information related to fertility but their website is particularly useful for IVF patients as it includes detailed information on all aspects of IVF treatment as well as information on statistics and success rates for U.S. infertility clinics.

These organizations are the largest and most established in the United States but there are also loads of smaller, often more specifically focused, organizations that depending on your diagnosis, preference and needs may be of interest to you. A great list of International and U.S.-based organizations focused on PCOS, endometriosis, infertility and cancer, Third-Party Reproduction, embryo donation, adoption, and more can be found on ASRM's website at www.reproductivefacts.org/Links.

GLOSSARY

AGI (ADJUSTED GROSS INCOME). A measure of income used to determine how much of your income is taxable. Adjusted gross income (AGI) is calculated as your gross income from taxable sources minus allowable deductions, such as unreimbursed business expenses, medical expenses, alimony, and deductible retirement-plan contributions.

AH (ASSISTED HATCHING). A micromanipulation procedure, in which an opening is made into the hard outer surface of an embryo with the use of chemicals, mechanical techniques, or lasers to assist in implantation to the uterine lining.

ART (ASSISTED REPRODUCTIVE TECHNOLOGY). Procedures to bring about conception without sexual intercourse.

BASELINE PELVIC ULTRASOUND. Ultrasound test to establish a reference point, used for comparison with any future ultrasounds. Used to determine the general position and condition of the pelvic structures and organs.

BETA OR HCG TEST. A blood test used to detect very early pregnancies.

BLASTOCYST (BLAST). A stage of embryonic development occurring about five days after fertilization. The embryo consists of two cell types, one that will form the placenta and one that will form the fetus and a central cavity.

BLIGHTED OVUM. An embryo that attaches itself to the uterine wall, but does not develop.

CELIAC DISEASE. An immune system reaction to eating gluten, a protein found in wheat, barley, and rye.

CERVIX. The lower, narrow end of the uterus that extends into the vagina, permitting sperm to enter and menstrual blood to exit. It produces mucus that helps the sperm to travel into the uterus.

CHEMICAL PREGNANCY. A pregnancy verified by lab tests but which results in an early miscarriage before gestation can be detected. The word "chemical" refers to the pregnancy being too early to confirm except through biochemical means.

CHROMOSOME. Contains the genetic information of an individual in the form of deoxyribonucleic acid (DNA).

CO-CULTURE/CULTURE MEDIUM. Used in IVF when living cells are added to manmade matter or a culture medium, usually to stimulate their growth and development.

COMPARATIVE GENOMIC HYBRIDIZATION (CGH). Genetic testing that can reveal whether an egg or embryo has the correct number of chromosomes (23 pairs, or 46 chromosomes) by taking a sample of DNA from a cell and evaluating the chromosome structure for extra or missing pieces.

CO-PAY. A type of insurance policy where the insured pays a specified amount of out-of-pocket expense for health-care services, such as doctor visits and prescriptions drugs, at the time the service is rendered, with the insurer paying the remaining costs.

CRYOPRESERVATION. A freezing process used to preserve eggs, embryos, sperm, and other types of tissue.

ECTOPIC PREGNANCY. Pregnancy located outside of the uterus, most commonly in a fallopian tube. Also called a *tubal pregnancy*.

EGG. The female reproductive cell. Also called oocyte or ovum, before it is released at ovulation.

EGG DONATION. Donation of an egg from one woman to another in hopes of the recipient becoming pregnant by in-vitro fertilization (IVF).

EGG RETRIEVAL. A procedure used to remove eggs from the ovaries' follicles for use in in-vitro fertilization (IVF).

EMBRYO. The fertilized egg (ovum) after it has begun the process of cell division.

EMBRYOLOGIST. A doctor who specializes in embryology.

EMBRYO TRANSFER. Placement of an embryo into the uterus of a woman after it has been created in a laboratory.

ENDOMETRIOSIS. A condition in which endometrial tissue, which normally lines the uterus, develops outside of the uterine cavity in abnormal locations, such as the ovaries, fallopian tubes, and/or abdominal cavity.

ESTRADIOL. A form of estrogen produced by the ovary. Estrogen concentrations in the blood are often measured during treatment cycles.

ESTROGEN. The main female sex hormone produced by the ovaries, responsible for the development of female sex characteristics. Largely responsible for stimulating the uterine lining to thicken during the first half of the menstrual cycle, in preparation for ovulation and possible pregnancy.

FALLOPIAN TUBES. A pair of hollow tubes attached, one on each side of the uterus, through which the egg travels from the ovary to the uterus.

FERTILIZATION. The successful union of the sperm and egg, resulting in cell division.

FET (FROZEN EMBRYO TRANSFER). The replacement of a fresh embryo with a cryo-preserved embryo in an IVF Cycle.

FIBROID. A non-cancerous, benign tumor of the uterine muscle wall. Also known as leiomyomas or myomas.

FISH (FLUORESCENCE IN-SITU HYBRIDIZATION). Screening of the embryo for familial genetic disorders. Can be used to count the number of chromosomes in an embryo and to visualize specific genes or portions of genes.

FOLLICULAR ASPIRATION. An ultrasound guided technique whereby a long, thin needle is passed through the vagina into the ovarian follicle. Suction is applied to accomplish retrieval of an egg.

FOLLICLE. A fluid-filled sac in the ovary containing the egg that is released at ovulation.

FSH (FOLLICLE-STIMULATING HORMONE). The pituitary hormone that stimulates follicle growth and the production of eggs in women, and sperm formation in men.

GENETIC TESTING. The use of specific tests to characterize the genetic status of an individual who is suspected to be at increased risk for an inherited disease. Also referred to as *genetic screening*, which is used to determine if a patient is at increased risk for passing on an inherited condition.

GESTATIONAL CARRIER. A woman who agrees to have a couple's fertilized egg (embryo) implanted in her uterus and carries the pregnancy for the couple. The carrier does not provide the egg and is therefore not biologically related to the child.

GnRH (GONADOTROPIN RELEASING HORMONE). The hormone produced and released by the hypothalamus that controls the pituitary gland's production and release of gonadotropins.

GN-RH AGONIST. Medications used to prevent premature ovulation which can come in two forms: A short-acting preparation administered over a few weeks and a long-acting preparation lasting for 1-3 months. Both types are typically administered in the early phases of an IVF cycle.

GN-RH ANTAGONIST. Another class of medications used to prevent premature ovulation, which are typically administered several days after stimulation.

GONADOTROPINS. Hormones, including FSH and LH, used for ovulation induction.

HCG (HUMAN CHORIONIC GONADOTROPIN). The hormone released naturally early in pregnancy. Also a medication used to trigger ovulation and progesterone production.

HPT (HOME PREGNANCY TEST). Pregnancy test that can be purchased over the counter.

HSG (HYSTEROSALPINGOGRAM). An x-ray examination of the uterus and fallopian tubes using a radio-opaque dye, used to check for malformations of the uterus or blocked fallopian tubes. Also called *hysterogram* or *tubogram*.

HYSTEROSCOPY. A procedure which allows examination of the inner cavity of the uterus through a fiber-optic telescope inserted through the vagina and cervical canal.

ICSI (INTRACYTOPLASMIC SPERM INJECTION). A micromanipulation technique used in IVF through which a single selected sperm is introduced directly into the cytoplasm of an egg.

IMPLANTATION. The moment an embryo or pre-embryo attaches itself to the uterine wall, resulting in pregnancy.

IRA (INDIVIDUAL RETIREMENT ACCOUNT). A savings account that allows individuals to direct pre-tax income toward investments that can grow tax-deferred (no capital gains or dividend income is taxed).

IRS (INTERNAL REVENUE SERVICE). A United States government agency that is responsible for the collection and enforcement of taxes.

IUI (INTRAUTERINE INSEMINATION). Technique which deposits washed sperm directly into the uterus, bypassing the cervix, and allowing the sperm to enter the fallopian tubes (where fertilization normally occurs).

IVF (IN-VITRO FERTILIZATION). A procedure where eggs are removed from the ovaries and mixed with sperm. Eggs that fertilize successfully become embryos and are transferred to the uterus in hopes that a pregnancy will result.

LH (LUTEINIZING HORMONE). The hormone that is released by the pituitary gland prior to ovulation which triggers ovulation and stimulates the corpus luteum to secrete progesterone.

MISCARRIAGE. The naturally occurring expulsion of a non-viable fetus and placenta from the uterus before the 20th week of pregnancy; also known as *spontaneous abortion* or *pregnancy loss*.

MOCK-TRANSFER. A preparatory procedure that helps to establish location and timing of embryo placement in an IVF transfer.

OB / GYN (OBstetrician GYNecologist). A physician whose specialty is health care for women.

OCPs (ORAL CONTRACEPTIVE PILLS). Medicines taken by mouth to prevent ovulation and pregnancy or to disguise symptoms of fertility problems, including irregular cycles, endometriosis, and ovarian cysts. Also called *birth control pills*.

OHSS (OVARIAN HYPERSTIMULATION SYNDROME). A condition that may result from excessive stimulation of the ovaries. It causes the ovaries to enlarge and create an overabundance of eggs.

OVARIES. The two small organs on either side of a woman's lower pelvis which produce ova, or eggs, and hormones.

OVARIAN CYSTS. Fluid-filled sacs that grow inside an ovary.

OVULATION. The release of a mature egg from its developing follicle in the ovary into the fallopian tubes.

PAP TEST. A procedure in which a physician scrapes cells from the cervix or vagina to check for cervical cancer, vaginal cancer, or abnormal changes that could lead to cancer. Also called a *pap smear*.

PCOS (POLYCYSTIC OVARIAN SYNDROME). A condition in which the ovaries contain many cystic follicles, which are associated with chronic anovulation and overproduction of androgens (male hormones).

(PGD) PRE-IMPLANTATION GENETIC TESTING. A test performed by an embryologist, in which one or two cells are removed from an embryo and screened for genetic abnormalities.

PROGESTERONE. The hormone produced during the second half (luteal phase) of a woman's cycle. It helps to thicken the lining of the uterus in preparation for implantation of a fertilized egg.

REPRODUCTIVE ENDOCRINOLOGIST (RE). An obstetrician-gynecologist who has completed additional training in reproductive endocrinology and is therefore qualified to manage imbalances in the complex hormonal reproductive system, including infertility and recurrent pregnancy loss.

SEMEN. The fluid, which contains a man's sperm, that is secreted from the testicles, seminal vesicles, and prostate during ejaculation.

SEMEN ANALYSIS. A laboratory test used to determine the amount and quality of a man's sperm and semen. Sperm may be measured by many factors including its count, volume, motility, morphology, and viability.

SEMEN COUNT. In a semen analysis: the number of sperm in the ejaculation or semen sample, usually given as the number of sperm per milliliter. Also called *sperm count*, *sperm concentration*, or *sperm density*.

SEMEN VOLUME. In a semen analysis, the measure of how much semen is present in one ejaculation or sample.

SEMEN MOTILITY. In a semen analysis, the measure of the percentage of sperm that can move forward normally. Also referred to as *sperm motility* or *forward progression*.

SEMEN MORPHOLOGY. In a semen analysis, the measure of the percentage of sperm that have a normal shape and size.

SHG (SONOHYSTEROGRAPHY). Imaging test of the uterus and uterine cavity using ultrasonography. Sterile saline is instilled into the uterine cavity with the purpose of detecting abnormalities of the uterus and endometrial (uterine) cavity.

SPERM. The male reproductive cell, or *gamete*.

SPERM WASHING. A technique used to separate sperm cells from the seminal fluid, resulting in a small volume of highly concentrated sperm used for ART treatments.

SPERM COUNT. The amount of sperm in a semen sample usually given as the number of sperm per milliliter. Also called *semen count*, *sperm concentration*, or *sperm density*.

THIRD-PARTY REPRODUCTION. The process by which a third person provides sperm or eggs, or in which another woman provides her uterus so that a woman can have a child through ART treatment.

THYROID DISEASE. Refers to disorders of the thyroid gland, which is an endocrine gland in the front of the neck that produces thyroid hormones to regulate the body's metabolism.

ULTRASOUND. A test that can either be performed abdominally or vaginally and that is used to produce pictures of internal organs by using high-frequency sound waves that are reflected off solid tissues to give an image of internal body structures. Used to detect and count follicle growth, to retrieve eggs, and to detect and monitor pregnancy. Can also be called a *sonography*.

UROLOGIST. A physician whose specialty is in urology, the branch of medicine that focuses on the surgical and medical diseases of the male and female urinary tract system and the male reproductive organs.